Praise for
Understanding Parkinson's Disease
A Self-Help Guide

"...Sympathetic guide to coping with a progressive,
disabling brain disorder. Kind, practical, and thorough..."
—*Kirkus Reviews*

"David Cram shares his experience and
...outlines sources for help and support."
—*Publisher's Weekly*

"[Dr. Cram] empathetically describes the aspects of Pd...
Quotes from Parkinson's patients enhance
the informative, authoritative text..."
—*Library Journal*

[Dr. Cram] discusses many pertinent drugs...
offers much practical advice...
and urges people to ask for help
without shyness or embarrassment.
—*Booklist*

"An outstanding resource.
Authoritative, readable, practical."
—*AgeVenture News Service*

Understanding Parkinson's Disease...

UNDERSTANDING
PARKINSON'S DISEASE

DAVID L. CRAM, M.D.

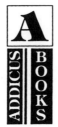

Addicus Books, Inc.
Omaha, Nebraska

An Addicus Nonfiction Book

ISBN 1-886039-40-2

Cover design by Jeff Reiner and Kelly Waggoner
Typography by Linda Dageforde

This book is not intended to serve as a substitute for a physician, nor does the author intend to give medical advice contrary to that of an attending physician.

Library of Congress Cataloging-in-Publication Data

Cram, David L. (David Lee), 1934-
    Understanding Parkinson's disease : a self-help guide / David L.
Cram.
      p.cm.
    "An Addicus nonfiction book."
    Includes bibliographical references and index.
    ISBN 1-886039-40-2 (alk. paper)
    1. Parkinson's disease—Popular works. I. Title.
RC382.C92   99-17981
616.8'3—dc21   CIP

Addicus Books, Inc.
Web site: www.AddicusBooks.com

*To my wife Elizabeth, who has stood by me
in my darkest hours*

Contents

Introduction

For those with a chronic, disabling neurological disorder such as Parkinson's disease, it is often hard to see a bright side to the adversity. Anger, self-pity, and fear may so cloud our perceptions, we choose despair over hope. We may feel so frightened we give up. We may feel like helpless victims, relying on others to perform even the most mundane tasks.

There is hope, even with a difficult disease like Parkinson's. New medications are available, and more are being developed all the time. Services are available to make your life and those of your caregivers easier. You can learn self-help strategies to help you feel better and remain physically active.

About now, you're probably grumbling, "What does he know about this dreadful disease?" I know because I have Parkinson's disease. I have felt anger, self-pity, fear, and despair. I have moved through those emotions and chosen to take charge of my disease and reclaim my life. You can, too.

When I was diagnosed with Parkinson's disease in 1989, my life changed forever. During the first few years, I felt alone, useless, and depressed. I no longer could do the things I loved. I was unwilling to accept that I had a progressive, disabling disease for which there is presently no cure. Being a doctor didn't help, either. During those dark times, all I could think about were people with severe Parkinson's disease whom I had encountered as a medical student. Vivid images of their stooped postures and shaking limbs haunted my thoughts. I sank further into depression and self-pity. I refused to attend Parkinson's support groups. I felt that if I could just deny reality, things would somehow be different. Not even the reassuring words of my friends and loved ones could alleviate my fear and loneliness. I was rapidly becoming a true victim of Parkinson's disease, broken in both body and spirit.

Despite my brooding in those early years, I continued to take the medications my doctors prescribed. One day I realized that the medications were working. My symptoms had lessened. I was able to do a number of things easily that I had not been able to do before. It also occurred to me that my disease was progressing much less rapidly than I had anticipated. I felt a glimmer of hope. Maybe I wasn't a victim after all. Perhaps I could fight this demon. At that moment I decided to reclaim my life. I resolved to learn all I could about Parkinson's disease. I decided to help myself instead of wallowing in self-pity. I would put my energy into exercises and self-help techniques that would help me feel better.

Once I decided to accept my fate and face the challenges it presented, incredible things began to happen. As if by magic, new and more effective drugs appeared in my life. I felt stronger and more empowered than at any time since my diagnosis. I tried out exercises and movements that helped me retain my flexibility and strength. I started reading everything I could about Parkinson's disease. I talked with others about how they coped, what worked for them.

Introduction

My search for a better life has become a crusade not only for myself, but hopefully for all who suffer from Parkinson's disease. This book contains the results of my search. May it help you feel better, cope more effectively, and face all of life's challenges with hope and optimism.

David L. Cram, M.D.

Adversity is not without comforts and hopes.
–Francis Bacon

1

A Self-Help Approach to Parkinson's Disease

If you or someone you love has been diagnosed with Parkinson's Disease (PD), it is easy to feel over-whelmed or believe there is nothing you can do. After all, PD is a chronic, progressive disease for which there is presently no cure. But, there *is* plenty you can do to improve your life or that of someone you love.

Self-help strategies can help improve the quality of life for those with PD. Self-help strategies can't cure the disease, but they can slow its progress and/or reduce the severity of symptoms. In addition, many new drugs can slow the progression of losses and eliminate many aggravating symptoms. The self-help techniques offered here can help you maintain your independence for as long as possible. Perhaps most importantly, they can help create a sense of well-being and serenity in your life.

What Is Self-Help?

Self-help is a positive approach to your condition that says, "I have power. I have responsibility. I can make a difference in my disease." There are four important elements of self-help:

1. Attitude
2. Knowledge
3. Partnership with your doctors
4. Taking action

Through education comes understanding. Through understanding comes compassion. Through compassion comes the best possible care.

Vicki, 45
Social worker

Attitude

Studies have repeatedly demonstrated that attitude can significantly affect one's health. For example, studies have shown that people who are hostile are more likely to suffer heart attacks. Our minds and bodies *are* connected. While eating right, exercising, reducing stress, and getting enough rest are all important, your attitude is perhaps the most essential element of self-help.

We do not yet know how attitude affects the physical aspects of PD. For instance, we do not know whether an upbeat attitude only lessens symptoms or actually slows the progression of the disease. However, we do know that a positive attitude can help improve the quality of your life. It *can* make you feel better. It can also help you take the self-help steps you need to keep feeling as good as you can for as long as you can.

Knowledge

Another essential tool of self-help is knowledge. It is important that you and your loved ones learn all you can about PD—what it is, what causes it, its symptoms, and treatment options. Stay abreast of the latest developments in research and treatment. Equipping yourselves with knowledge will reduce your fears and enable you to make the best-informed medical choices.

Partnership with Your Doctors

Self-help does not mean doing everything by and for yourself. Because you have a serious, progressive disease, your doctors must play a major role in your care. The old model of healthcare presumed that the doctor had all the power. He/she made all the decisions concerning your medical care. By contrast, the self-help model acknowledges that you are an active partner with your doctors in your healthcare. Self-help comes with responsibilities. For instance, your doctors must select the right medicine in the correct dosage for your symptoms. Your job is to take the right amount of medication on time, to keep track of your symptoms and side effects, and to let the doctors know how the medication is working and any problems you may be having with it.

Before I knew much about PD, I was very frightened. Once I started learning as much as I could, my fears lessened. Knowing more gives me a better sense of control.

Perry
Age 67

Taking Action

Taking action means doing the things that make you feel better, help slow the disability, and keep you as independent as possible for as long as possible. You can use specific self-help strategies to improve your diet, to take your medications on time in the right amounts, to reduce stress in your life, and to get adequate rest. I will discuss each of these strategies further in the coming chapters.

By adopting a positive, upbeat attitude, equipping yourself with knowledge, partnering with your doctors, and taking action, you will give yourself the best possible chance at living better with PD.

What Is Parkinson's Disease?

PD is a progressive, disabling brain disorder. Doctors often call it a *motor system disorder.* PD occurs when brain cells, or *neurons*, decline and cause a deficiency in the chemical brain messenger *dopamine.* Dopamine helps the nervous system control muscle activity. The low supply of dopamine causes the major symptoms of PD.

Major Symptoms

Tremor

The trembling can affect the hands, arms, legs, jaw, and face. The classic PD tremor is a rhythmic back-and-forth movement of the thumb and forefinger, sometimes described as "pill rolling." The tremor usually begins in the hand but may also begin in the foot or jaw. About seventy-five percent of people with PD develop tremor; in the early stages of the disease, the tremor affects only one side of the body. Approximately twenty-five percent never develop significant tremor.

Stiffness or rigidity

For the body to move smoothly, opposing sets of muscles must alternately relax and contract. In a person with PD, muscles of the limbs and trunk may remain constantly tense and contracted. This may cause aching, stiffness, weakness, and jerky movements.

Slowness of movement

Called *bradykinesia,* slowing down is an unpredictable and frustrating symptom of PD. One moment, a person moves easily. The next, he/she needs help. Simple tasks such as dressing that were once performed easily may become difficult and time-consuming.

Education is the key. I go to every support group meeting I can and read whatever I can get my hands on. Everything I have learned has helped me care for my wife and myself in some way.

Joe
Age 81

Impaired balance and coordination

This symptom may prevent someone with PD from performing certain motor functions, making him/her fall easily or have a stooped posture. These symptoms tend to worsen over time. Eventually, there may be difficulty walking, talking, or completing otherwise simple tasks.

Other Possible Symptoms

Depression

It is common, especially early in the disease, for a person to develop depression. Drugs used to treat PD symptoms sometimes worsen depression.

Emotional Changes

Insecurity and fear are often secondary symptoms of PD. A person may fear he/she can't cope with new situations and will refuse to travel or socialize.

Memory Loss/Slow Thinking

While reasoning remains clear, it may be harder for someone with PD to remember or come up with solutions as quickly as he/she once did.

Problems Swallowing/Chewing

In the later stages of PD, the muscles are less efficient, making it difficult to swallow or chew. Fortunately, medications can usually solve these difficulties.

Changes in Speech

One with PD may experience changes in speech: rapid speech, slurred or repeated words, hesitation in speaking, or speaking too softly or in a monotone. Speech therapy can often help.

Urinary problems/constipation

Some individuals with PD may have difficulty controlling his/her bowels and bladder and suffer constipation. Changes in diet, exercise, and drinking plenty of fluids can often alleviate constipation.

I remember the moment I knew something was wrong. A friend took me country western line dancing. I was having a great time, when my friend asked me, "Why don't you smile?" But I thought I was standing there smiling. I felt confused and frustrated.

Katherine
Age 57

Oily/Dry Skin

It is common to develop oily or dry skin or facial rashes. One may also sweat excessively and/or experience feelings of heat or cold. Medication and standard skin treatments can usually alleviate these problems.

Difficulty Sleeping

Those with PD may have restless sleep, nightmares, and problems staying asleep at night. As a result, he/she may feel drowsy during the day. Difficulty sleeping may be a symptom of PD and/or a side effect of the drugs used to treat symptoms of the disease.

I was scared when I heard my diagnosis. I didn't know what it meant or what the next step was. Taking the initiative to learn about the disease has lessened my fears and has taken the mystery out of things.

Jeanne
Age 66

Handwriting Problems

It is not uncommon for someone with PD to notice changes in his/her handwriting; it often becomes small and crowded.

Backache

Back pain is often accompanied by poor posture.

Changes in Expression

Others may notice that a loved one with PD has less facial expression. He/she may smile less and have what is called a "mask-like face." One may also blink less, giving the appearance of staring; this results from the loss of automatic muscle movements.

Freezing

In these incidents, PD causes one to suddenly stop or "freeze." It's as if someone hit an "off" switch and stopped you in your tracks. The "off" period usually lasts only a few seconds or minutes.

Stages of PD: How the Disease Progresses

PD affects people differently. In some people, the disease progresses quickly. In others, it progresses quite slowly. Some become quite disabled from the symptoms. Others experience only minor symptoms.

For most, there is a subtle "presymptomatic" phase, which may begin four to six years before more obvious PD symptoms. A person may feel tired or generally unwell. He/she may feel a bit shaky or have trouble getting out of a chair. Other subtle, early symptoms may include:

- slight weakness in an extremity
- stiffness in one leg when walking
- slight trembling
- mood changes
- changes in posture
- decreased sense of smell
- memory problems
- dizziness
- handwriting problems
- changes in speech
- muscle and joint pains

Often the disease begins with a small tremor in one finger that comes and goes. Over time, the tremor may become more frequent and spread to the entire arm. Stiffness or rigidity in the arm may follow. Simple tasks such as buttoning clothes may become difficult. With time, the leg on the affected side may become stiff and rigid, harder to move.

In many cases these changes are so subtle or gradual, a person doesn't really notice them. Often family or friends are the first to notice.

My initial reaction was relief when my doctor told me I had Parkinson's Disease —I had thought a I had a brain tumor. I didn't know what PD was, which shows the need for public education about this disease.

Robert
Age 64

It was my wife who first noticed the changes—the slowness of my movements, the shuffling of my feet, my stooped posture. When I came home from work, I felt very tired. I began to go to bed earlier and earlier. Even after a good night's sleep, I never felt rested.

After a time, even my patients noticed the changes. A well-meaning patient said to me, "Dr. Cram, you look like an old man. Put your shoulders back and straighten up." Her comments stabbed me like a knife.

As the years pass, the symptoms progress. The tremor and the rigidity may spread to both sides of the body. Movement may become slower. One's facial expression becomes less animated.

Especially in older people, it is easy to see how stiff limbs, slow movement, and a shuffling gait may be confused with normal, age-related changes. Many people with PD and their loved ones dismiss the early symptoms as "old age." Sometimes the fatigue and lack of facial expression leads to an incorrect diagnosis of depression. Since the symptoms often progress slowly over many years, it may take quite some time before they interfere enough to prompt one to seek a medical diagnosis.

Doctors classify PD symptoms by stages. For instance, your doctor may say, "You have stage 1 Parkinson's Disease." What does this mean?

Stage 1

- Signs and symptoms appear only on one side of the body.
- Symptoms are mild.

- Symptoms may be inconvenient, but they are not disabling.
- Usually a tremor is present in only one limb.
- Friends and other loved ones have noticed changes in posture, movement, and in facial expression.

Stage 2

- Symptoms appear on both sides of the body.
- Symptoms cause minimal disability.
- Posture and gait are affected.

Stage 3

- Body movements are slowed significantly.
- Symptoms cause moderately severe problems with normal functioning.

Stage 4

- Symptoms are severe.
- The individual can still walk, but only to a limited extent.
- There is rigidity and slowness of movement.
- One is no longer able to live alone.

Neurologists include a fifth stage in which the debilitation requires a patient to be confined to a bed or wheelchair. For many patients, early self-help and drug therapy may delay this stage to very late in the disease or even prevent it.

Who Gets PD?

You may be asking, "Why did I get PD?" No one really knows. But you're not alone. According to the National Institutes of Health, one-half million Americans have PD. Between 20,000 and 50,000 new cases are diagnosed each year. More people suffer from PD than from multiple sclerosis, muscular dystrophy, and amyotrophic lateral sclerosis (Lou Gehrig's disease) combined. The average age for the onset of PD is sixty-one, but the disease may strike at any age. However, only about one-third of all new PD cases occur among persons under fifty.

What Causes PD?

Unfortunately, doctors do not know what causes the brain's neurons to die or become impaired. Many studies have failed to reveal a virus as the cause of PD. In a few cases, PD-like symptoms have resulted from repeated blows to the head or from carbon monoxide poisoning. Recently, several young people developed Parkinsonism after taking a heroin that contained the drug *MPTP*, a heroin derivative. However, for most people with classic PD, doctors do not know the cause of their disease. Scientists have a number of theories.

> *I'm fortunate that my PD has progressed slowly. I've also responded well to medications. This past year I went to Europe and Mexico.*
> *David*
> *Age 64*

Oxidative Damage

Some researchers suggest that *free radicals*, molecules generated by normal chemical reactions in the body, may damage or kill nerve cells and lead to PD symptoms. Free radicals react with other molecules in a process called *oxidation*. This process is believed to damage tissues, including neurons.

Environmental Toxins

Other scientists believe external or internal toxins may destroy the dopamine-messenger neurons. Some suggest exposure to pesticides, carbon monoxide, heavy metals, drug reactions, or toxins in the food supply may cause such damage.

Accelerated Aging

Another theory proposes that PD symptoms occur when the normal, age-related wearing away of dopamine-producing neurons speeds up. The reason for this accelerated aging is not known.

Genetic Factors

A relatively new theory suggests the tendency to develop PD may be inherited. Some families have multiple cases of PD, but these are rare. Without an obvious family history, the risk of your offspring developing PD is thought not to be a reason for concern.

Although doctors do not know what causes it, a PD-like state may be caused by a number of drugs. For instance, some tranquilizers (haloperidol, thioridazine, chlorpromazine) and high-blood-pressure drugs that contain resperine may interfere with the dopamine in the brain and cause symptoms of PD. Fortunately, parkinsonism caused from drugs is usually reversible. When the individual stops taking the drugs, the symptoms commonly disappear. Some people with hardened, narrowed arteries (*arteriosclerosis*) who have suffered strokes develop PD-like symptoms. In such cases, an accurate diagnosis of PD may prove difficult. In recent years, doctors have seen PD in people between the ages of twenty-one and thirty-nine. In such early onset of PD, symptoms tend to progress more slowly, but certain side effects from the drug levodopa may appear earlier. Less than 10 percent of people with PD develop early onset.

> *Success is not measured by what you achieved but rather what you never gave up trying to do. I never give in to limitations. I thrive on that challenge.*
>
> *Daisy*
> *Age 69*

How Is PD Diagnosed?

In the early stages, PD may be difficult to diagnose. Early symptoms may be vague and seemingly unrelated. They may mysteriously come and go. As mentioned earlier, PD symptoms may be confused with normal, age-related changes.

Diagnosing PD may be difficult even for a neurologist familiar with the disease. There are no blood or lab tests that can definitively diagnose PD. Doctors diagnose it with a neurological examination that includes looking at the type and severity of symptoms, especially the three classic PD symptoms: tremors, rigidity, and slowness of movement.

As with anything, being a success is hard work. I've dedicated my life to making myself well and am making tremendous progress. Setting goals and achieving them is truly a euphoric feeling.

Jim
Age 56

Get a second and even a third opinion, if needed. If only one doctor says you have PD, it is easy to say, "That doctor doesn't know what he/she is talking about." But if two or three doctors confirm the diagnosis, it is harder to deny.

Be realistic about your symptoms. How long have you felt not quite yourself? Make a list of all the symptoms you have noticed. Then read the list over. Do you have any of the "classic" PD symptoms—tremor, slowness of movement, or stiffness?

Ask friends and family for their opinions. What symptoms have they noticed?

Give yourself time. It is difficult to accept that you have a chronic, progressive disease. Take your time. Try to gradually take a new view of things.

A physician may suggest a trial of antiparkinson drugs, usually levodopa. If a patient's symptoms improve with the drug, PD is likely the diagnosis. If he/she does not get better with the drug, the problem may be something else. The doctor may also want to conduct scans of the brain. Although neither *computed tomography* (CT) nor *magnetic resonance imaging* (MRI) can diagnose PD, these brain-imaging tools can rule out other diseases that may produce PD-like symptoms.

3

The Emotional Side of Parkinson's Disease

Long-term, chronic ailments such as PD can disrupt family life, strain marriages, alienate friends and colleagues, and drain hard-earned financial resources. Learning you have PD can be devastating. You may feel angry, guilty, afraid, and resentful. You may deny you have the disease, withdraw, or become depressed. One of the most important things to know is that these feelings and reactions are normal. Most people diagnosed with PD have experienced some or all of them at one time or another.

There are no right or wrong, good or bad reactions to such a diagnosis. No one can tell you how to react. Your reaction to the disease and how you cope with it will determine the shape and color of your life, and to a lesser degree, the lives of your loved ones.

Overcoming Denial

PD tends to sneak up on people, coming on imperceptibly in small degrees. Before your diagnosis, you likely knew you were not quite yourself. You may have dismissed your symptoms, denying anything was seriously wrong for as long as you could. This reaction is normal and very common. Denial is a form of self-protection. We never want to admit there's something seriously wrong. Before your diagnosis, you probably found yourself torn between denial of any problem and fear and worry about what the problem might be. As your symptoms progressed and you experienced more physical limitations, the mental strain and worry probably became even more severe.

Just because patients are disabled doesn't mean that they are unable. Yes, there are some limitations, but they can still accomplish daily tasks by simply making accommodations.

Mary Ellen, 38
Occupational therapist

I refused to believe I might be developing a neurological disease. I didn't rush out and seek medical advice. But as my symptoms progressed, there came a time when I had to face reality. One day, I told my wife to draw a chalk line on the patio. "If I can't walk this straight line without falling off," I said, "I'll go for a neurological exam tomorrow." I failed the test.

If you're like most people, you find the diagnosis of PD both a shock and a relief. You have just been told that you have a progressive, disabling disease. Yet there is some relief in at last being able to put a diagnosis on your vague symptoms. Suddenly your future looks uncertain. Questions fill your mind: What will I be able to do? Is it possible to continue working? Can I still function as a parent or partner? What kind of medical bills will I have to deal with?

A neurologist gave me the news in August 1989. I was fifty-five years old, a doctor with a busy and successful medical practice. The diagnosis hit me like a ton of bricks. My mind was a jumble of conflicting thoughts and emotions: "How could this be? I'm healthy. I'm a doctor. I have a lot of things to do. This isn't happening."

My doctor tried to reassure me that, with today's medications, people with PD often can live a normal life span and usually die from some unrelated health problem. I barely heard his words.

Physical symptoms forced me to stop working, but they didn't keep me from living. My wife and I bought a camper and have visited all fifty states.

Henry
Age 63

It is not uncommon even after the doctor says you have PD to deny it, to refuse to accept it. However, denying the disease expends a great deal of energy and causes anxiety. Trying to hide your symptoms may cause you embarrassment and isolation. As long as you deny the disease, you are an unwitting victim of it. The sooner you accept your condition, the sooner you can begin coping with it and living your life.

Conquering Unfounded Fears

You may have seen friends, relatives, or acquaintances who suffered from PD before there were effective medications like l-dopa. These images may be terribly frightening, causing you to believe that PD is a severely disabling and untreatable disease.

Fortunately, these notions are inconsistent with today's medicine. Many of the symptoms of PD can be successfully treated with medications.

There are several ways to combat unfounded fears and to prevent your imagination from causing you undue distress.

Find a doctor you can work with. Look for someone who will talk with you about your fears and concerns.

Learn all you can about the disease. See the recommended reading list in Resources, at the end of this book.

Talk about your fears with your doctor, your family, and supportive friends. It helps to "air" your fears. When you bring them into the light, they appear much smaller.

Join a PD support group. Aside from providing camaraderie and moral support, members of such groups can give information about the latest treatments, referrals to physicians, and practical tips on how to cope.

Talk with a mental health professional. If these strategies aren't enough to keep your fears from overwhelming you, talk with a mental health professional such as a neuropsychologist.

> *The word limitation can be singular or plural. A single limitation imposed on you doesn't mean it's time to limit all aspects of your life. Accept limitations and run wild with your freedoms.*
>
> *Bill*
> *Age 49*

Regaining a Sense of Control

A common reaction to a diagnosis of PD is "Why me?" Suddenly your life seems dangerously out of control. As much as we try to control the events of our lives, there are times when we are helpless to control certain forces. You can't do anything about a slick, icy patch on the road. Nor can you do anything about a mechanical failure on an airplane you're flying. Nor can you do anything about the fact that the dopamine in your brain is depleted.

Feeling out of control can make you feel like a victim. It can deplete your energy and your motivation and make you feel needlessly dependent on others. The good news is, you can regain a sense of control in your life.

While you can't do anything about having PD, there is plenty you can do about how it affects your life. Just as learning about PD can help control your fears, it can also give you a sense of control. Here are a few other tips for regaining your equilibrium:

Create your own definition of success. Keep in mind that you don't have to do it all to be successful. Shining in just one area, perhaps by making a difference in another person's life, can make you a success.
Wendy, 33
Rehabilitation counselor

Become an active participant in your healthcare. Don't just accept what your doctor says. Ask questions. If you don't understand, ask until you do. Offer suggestions.

Stay as independent as possible. Some people react to chronic illness by becoming increasingly dependent on others. Eventually, they may become totally helpless, not from the disease itself but from their emotional reactions to it. Instead, do as much for yourself as you can, asking for help only when you really need it.

Make a plan for yourself. Work closely with your doctor to develop an effective treatment plan. Make a list of all the things you can do to help yourself such as exercising, eating right, managing stress, and taking your medicine on time.

Reclaiming a Sense of Self

"Who am I?" you may wonder. Be assured that you are more than your disease. You may not be able to do all the things you did before PD, but you are still a valuable individual. Here are some tips for bolstering your internal defenses and reclaiming a strong sense of self.

Learn to accept help. It is difficult to be dependent on others, but your condition will make you unable to do certain things. You *will* need help. Learn to accept this increased level of dependence without losing your dignity.

Learn to cope with negative responses from others. Sometimes, you will have to deal with unkind responses from others, especially strangers. If you experience staring, hostility, pity, rejection, or other negative responses, try to chalk it up to others' lack of knowledge about this complex disease.

Talk with others about how they cope. Others with chronic diseases have walked the same road and know how it feels. Talking and sharing feelings, thoughts, and ideas with them can help you feel less alone and less different.

Recall your past successes. That doesn't mean dwelling on the past or grieving for what was. Just keep in mind your past contributions, honors, and successes. Those memories can bolster you when you are feeling down.

Focus on small victories. It's not the huge successes that count over time, but dozens of small ones. Set goals and keep track of your successes. You might consider keeping a written or taped journal of your victories that you can review to keep your spirits up.

Avoid lashing out. Sometimes you will feel angry about your disease. Avoid putting your anger on others, especially loved ones and caregivers.

Avoid destructive behaviors. Some people turn to drugs and alcohol to numb the pain of difficult challenges like chronic illness. These are only temporary fixes and ultimately will make your disease even more difficult to deal with.

Dumping Depression

Depression is common among people with PD. Experts estimate that as many as 40 percent of people with PD suffer from depression. Depression is different and more serious from "the blues" that most of us feel from time to time. The symptoms of depression include:

- depressed mood
- diminished interest or loss of pleasure in all or almost all activities
- weight loss or weight gain when not dieting
- inability to sleep or oversleeping
- restlessness (agitation) or slowing down so that it is noticeable to others
- fatigue or loss of energy
- feelings of worthlessness
- diminished ability to think or concentrate
- recurrent thoughts of suicide or death

If you have a depressed mood and/or loss of interest and at least four of the other symptoms during the same two-week period, you are likely depressed. While most people with PD experience only mild depression, a few suffer moderate or even severe depression.

Depression may be caused by biochemical changes in the brains of some people with PD. Studies have revealed that people who suffer from depression have reduced levels of serotonin, a brain chemical believed to play a major role in the regulation of mood. Doctors call this biochemical imbalance in the brain *endogenous depression*. It can be life-threatening if not treated.

Medications used to treat PD may also cause depression. Usually, when depression is caused by PD medications, it starts with anxiety, restlessness, or worry in the first two weeks after beginning the medication. This period may be followed by sleeplessness and/or mood swings for several weeks. Symptoms usually peak after five or six weeks as the body adapts to the medication and the depression begins to lift. If you believe your depression is related to the medications you are taking, talk with your doctor. Perhaps your medication or dosage can be changed.

Because some of the symptoms of depression—fatigue, slow movement, reduced facial expression, insomnia, difficulty concentrating—are also PD symptoms, PD-related depression is often confused or misdiagnosed. In the early stages, depression might mask PD symptoms. Later on, PD symptoms may hide depression.

Sitting around the house in my pajamas did nothing for my self-esteem. One day I realized I have the ability to do so much more. Give yourself time to sort through all your emotions after being diagnosed, then get on with your life.
Agnes
Age 71

If you have symptoms of depression, it is important to have them treated. Your doctor can prescribe antidepressant medication that can help. The same medication may also alleviate other

PD symptoms. In addition to medication, there are many other things you can do to lift your spirits.

Get active. Physical activity releases *endorphins,* the body's own natural mood elevators. If you cannot do a task because you're tired or "off," do something else. The key is to remain as physically and mentally active as possible.

Identify your goals. To keep depressive feelings from overwhelming you, set small, specific goals that are realistic and attainable. Establish a time frame for each goal. Set goals in all areas of your life: physical activity, employment, social activities, spiritual growth, and recreational activities like crafts that will help tune your motor skills. Your list of goals may look something like this:

- Exercise at least fifteen minutes every day.
- Attend a PD support group once a week.
- Take a class on the Internet this month.

Avoid self-criticism. It's easy to be critical of yourself when you are feeling depressed. When you hear that inner voice giving negative messages such as "I'm too slow" or "I used to be able to do this, but now I can't," refocus attention on positive accomplishments. Replace negative messages with positive ones: "I do my job well," "I'm an excellent parent," and "I have a good relationship with my family."

Stay connected with others. It's not unusual for people in the early stages of PD to feel embarrassed about their symptoms, especially tremors. They may believe having a chronic illness, especially one that makes it difficult or awkward to move around, makes them social outcasts. To avoid embarrassment, they may withdraw from others and stay away from their usual social and recreational activities. Isolation may deepen feelings of depression. Staying connected with others is vitally important to your mental and emotional health. Seize the opportunity to interact with others by participating in church activities, entertaining, taking classes, visiting friends, volunteering, and attending support-group meetings.

Talk about your feelings. Share your thoughts, feelings, fears, concerns, hopes, and dreams with friends and loved ones. Don't be afraid to talk about your feelings of fear, loneliness, embarrassment, anger, and frustration. You may be surprised how sharing your inner feelings will deepen your relationships.

Try counseling. If these strategies don't provide enough relief, try talking with a mental health counselor for additional support.

Reducing Stress

Stress can often make PD symptoms, especially tremors, worse. While researchers have ruled out stress as a cause of PD, stress can trigger symptoms or magnify them. It is important to effectively manage stress.

Identify sources of stress. Different things are stressful to different people. Even pleasant situations may be stressful. For many with PD, especially those newly diagnosed, social situations may cause anxiety and worsen symptoms, causing even more stress. The key is not to avoid social situations and become isolated, but to evaluate such situations and decide how you can make changes to reduce the stress. Make a list of those things that cause you stress.

Plan changes to reduce stress and act on your plan. For example, what if the last time you had lunch with friends several pieces of your lunch ended up on the floor because you had dif-

> *Humor is everywhere; don't be afraid to laugh at it. Laughter is a good release of tension, anxiety and worries. It really is the best medicine.*
>
> *Michelle, 26*
> *RN*

ficulty cutting the meat? You may have felt humiliated and embarrassed. When your friend calls to schedule another luncheon, your first thought is to decline the invitation and avoid another potentially embarrassing situation. Instead, ask yourself, "How could I do this differently? How could I accommodate my condition and still enjoy lunching with my friends?" One solution would be to order a dish that does not require the fine motor skills to cut meat. Another solution would be to ask the waiter to cut up your portion into bite-sized pieces before bringing it to the table. Or you could ask your friend if he/she would mind cutting your entree for you.

When I realized that my stubbornness hurt my children just as much as it hurt me, I stopped pushing them away and accepted their assistance. Now I enjoy the time we spend together; we've grown closer.

Ben
Age 75

Adjust your expectations. Pushing yourself to perform mentally and physically exactly as you once did may bring on undue anxiety.

Reprioritize. A serious illness forces you to reevaluate your life. What's really important to you? Is it closing one more sale, or spending more time with your granddaughter? Is it earning more money, or volunteering with a cause you feel passionate about? Only you can decide what's most important. Be aware that such self-examination may result in your changing jobs or not keeping the house spotless every day. Your new priorities may help bring you closer to your true self and what makes you happy.

Set goals. Make your goals realistic, so that they are attainable, and challenging, so that they make you "stretch" just a bit. Again, take time to set goals in all areas of your life: social, spiritual, physical, financial, and so on. Establish both weekly goals and longer-term goals.

Plan your time to avoid stressful deadlines. Many of us are caught in a time crunch. We often rush, barely getting to appointments on time. Allow more time for everything. Whenever possible set approximate times for appointments so that if you're running behind you won't feel as if you're late.

Get plenty of sleep. Plan your schedule whenever possible so that you get extra rest after a particularly busy day. If your lifestyle allows it, schedule a refreshing nap in the afternoon. Research has shown that short afternoon naps (less than forty-five minutes) can make one more relaxed, refreshed, and alert.

Limit caffeine. It can make you jittery. Coffee, black tea, cola, and other items may contain caffeine. Try drinking decaf varieties or limit yourself to one caffeinated cup a day. Avoid drinking caffeinated beverages before retiring for the night.

Get organized. Develop systems to help you find things easily. Put items in the same place every day. For instance, putting your keys and wallet in one place will help avoid the anxiety of not being able to find them, especially when you're rushed.

Ask for help. This may be one of the hardest things to do. No one likes to feel dependent. But you will need to ask family and friends for assistance with some activities. Asking for help not only allows you to be vulnerable and open to others, it allows them to give you the gift of help. At first it may feel difficult, but over time such interdependence may bring people closer together.

Practice deep breathing. Sit quietly with your eyes closed. To the count of four, breathe in deeply, filling your lungs and your abdomen. Then slowly release it. Repeat for five or six breaths.

Progressively relax. Sit or lie in a quiet place where you won't be disturbed. Starting at your head, tense and then release groups of muscles. Work down your entire body, progressively tensing and releasing muscles. Once you've tensed and released all the way to your feet, sit quietly for several minutes.

Meditate. Take a meditation class. Or try this simple meditation technique. Sit quietly with your eyes closed, breathing normally. Each time you inhale, think the word "one" (or "peace," "calm," or "om"). As thoughts come up, let them go and gently refocus on your word and your breathing. Continue for ten to fifteen minutes. At first, you may be bothered by many thoughts, or "monkey mind" as some call it. Don't worry. With practice, you will find that you are better able to quiet your mind and enjoy the peaceful silence. Take a meditation break in the morning and in the early evening, or whenever you are feeling tired or in need of a break.

> *When I decided to regain my independence, the progress I made was unbelievable. It's amazing how the power of the mind can push the body to the maximum.*
>
> *Margaret*
> *Age 54*

Practice yoga. Yoga can help calm your mind and keep your body more limber. Many postures involve gentle stretching, strengthening, and deep breathing.

Explore biofeedback. This involves learning to control your own body functions with visual or auditory stimulation. You will first have to learn the techniques from a physician or a biofeedback technician. Once you have learned them, they can help you feel more in control of your stress level and your body.

Relax with guided imagery. There are hundreds of tapes you can buy or check out from the library that combine relaxing sounds and/or music with instructions for an imaginary "trip." For instance, guided imagery might involve visualizing yourself walking by the sea on a beautiful, cloudless day and feeling the wind caress your skin. Or it might involve lying in a green meadow where you can smell the flowers, hear the gentle twitter of birds, and feel the sun warming your body. Once you become accustomed to using these tapes, you will be able to visualize on your own and take a little "mental vacation" whenever the need arises.

Telling Others about Your Disease

Telling others about your PD may cause anxiety and stress. When should you tell? Whom should you tell? Should you tell your employer? What about your children or grandchildren? How much should you tell? There are no right or wrong answers to these questions. Some people opt to tell everyone they know to avoid questions and curious looks. Others choose to tell only those closest to them until symptoms become evident. You must find your own answers to these questions.

Communicate openly and truthfully with your family. They will appreciate it and you will feel better too. Also be honest with friends and neighbors; it will prevent them from trying to guess what is wrong.

Lisa
Age 39

One thing is certain. Attempting to hide your disease, especially as symptoms worsen, will only lead to increased anxiety. This, in turn, may worsen your symptoms. Experts have found that those who are able to accept their disease and tell others about it cope best.

Keep in mind that PD affects not only you but all those close to you. Effectively coping with and treating PD requires the assistance, understanding, and cooperation of all those in your social network. Keeping it a secret just makes it harder to begin the process of adjusting and coping with your disease. Below are some general tips about telling family, friends, coworkers, acquaintances, employers, and others about your condition.

Be direct and honest. Once you decide who to tell, there's no use trying to "sugar-coat" the situation. At work, be sure to talk with your supervisor before telling coworkers. The grapevine has a way of passing information to those you least want to know.

Don't wait too long. If your symptoms are noticeable, others may talk behind your back. Often, they will come up with the wrong diagnosis.

> *I go to every support group meeting I can and read everything about PD. The knowledge I have gained helps me understand what my husband is going through.*
>
> *Joyce*
> *Age 59*

Let people know how they can help. Many people will genuinely want to help. Your needs will change. Be ready to let others know about your changing needs.

Give others a place to learn about PD. Some people, especially those close to you, may need to learn more about PD. Finding out about the disease can reassure them that there are many people with PD who are living full and active lives. An abundance of literature is available from national PD organizations, several of which are listed in the resource section of this book. You'll also find information on the world wide web and in local libraries.

Talking with Your Partner

When you have a chronic illness, your partner is affected almost as completely as you are. Often, he/she is present when you receive a PD diagnosis. If not, it's important that you share the information with your mate as soon as possible.

> *My wife was away on a business trip when I went to the neurologist's office and received my diagnosis. I phoned her right away. She took the news more calmly and more rationally than I did. But, then, she always was better at dealing with strong emotions.*

Any long-term illness can strain a marriage or long-term relationship to the breaking point. If the relationship is already on shaky ground, a PD diagnosis may be the final blow. Your partner may not be able or willing to endure the realities of coping with a long-term illness. He/she may deny its reality. Your partner may feel angry or resentful that major aspects of the relationship may change, including traditional roles. Or he/she may become fearful and overprotective, always wanting to "take care" of you. Although these responses are perfectly normal and quite common, none fosters the work of coping with PD. If you're more fortunate and have a stable, loving relationship, the diagnosis of PD will test but not destroy your partnership. Instead, over time, it may even bring you closer together.

Facing your partner's reactions is one of the most difficult aspects of PD. Nevertheless, it is important not to let your mate's responses aggravate your symptoms. Here are some strategies for helping your mate cope:

Be honest about your condition. Don't try to "soft-pedal" your prognosis to spare your partner. Likewise, don't try to make it more serious than it is. You are in this together, so both of you deserve to be fully and honestly informed.

Accept his/her reactions. Remember, there are no "right" ways for a partner to respond.

Reassure. Let your mate know that, with treatment, most people with PD live long and productive lives and that most, if not all, symptoms can be controlled.

Remain as independent as possible. Ask for help when you need it, but don't become overly dependent upon your mate. Caregiving is difficult. Your partner has enough to do without you becoming more dependent than is necessary.

Encourage your mate to fully participate with your healthcare team. This will help both of you feel as if you're in this together and help regain a sense of control.

Learn about the disease together. Both partners should gather materials about PD and learn all you can about the disease.

Encourage your partner to attend caregiver support groups. Many communities offer support groups for partner-caregivers in which they can talk about their feelings, get practical tips for coping, and feel less alone.

Support your partner's outside interests and contacts. It is important for your mate to develop and maintain outside interests such as community groups, sports, visiting friends, church/synagogue groups, and classes. Your mate will feel less stressed and will become a better caregiver if he/she has interests outside of you and your condition.

Honestly discuss your financial picture. One of the biggest fears a partner faces when the other person becomes ill is the loss of income. Sit down and take a realistic look at your financial situation. Review your health insurance. Develop a realistic budget. Can you cut some expenses to save money? If needed, check out federal, state, and county sources of financial assistance.

Assess your support system. Who else in your circle of family and friends can you count on for help? Full-time partner-care-givers need help and respite. If your partner can't drive you to the doctor, who else can?

Talk, talk, talk. Close communication is key to coping effectively together with PD and maintaining close ties. Good communication can be the difference between a partnership that weathers this latest storm or one that becomes overwhelmed.

Talking with Children

At some point children too need to be told. Give consideration to how you will tell them.

At first, my wife and I decided not to tell my thirteen-year-old stepson. He has always been very sensitive and tuned in to me, and I was afraid he wouldn't take it well. As my disease progressed, he noticed my symptoms and began to ask about them. When I told him, I tried to sound confident and reassure him. I think this made it easier for him to accept my condition.

Show patients that they are special, loved and wanted in the family. Include them in family affairs. Constantly praise them. Remind them how far they have come. Celebrate milestones.

Betsy, 51
Counselor

Use age-appropriate language. Too much or too little information given in a way that feels scary or threatening may stimulate a child's fantasies and fears. To a young child you might say, "Grandmother has a sickness that makes her hands shake." To a teenager you might say, "I have a nerve problem that makes my hands tremble." Don't speculate about the future, what might happen. As the condition progresses, you may need to give more information.

Encourage the child to ask questions. Kids are wonderful at asking direct questions, especially if you let them know it's all right to talk about your condition. "Why don't you stand up straight, Grandpa?" "Why don't you smile, Mommy?" "Why is your voice so soft, Aunt Mary?"

Let children share their concerns. When fears are suppressed, they may grow out of proportion. Create an open atmosphere that lets children express their fears, anxieties, and concerns about your condition.

Reassure. Let children know that your condition isn't fatal and that it isn't contagious. Often children are afraid they might "catch" others' health problems. Let older children know that most evidence suggests that PD is not an inherited disease. Also reassure them that you didn't get the disease because of anything they or anyone else did or did not do.

Keep the tone light and conversational. If you cry or let your anxiety show, children may worry unnecessarily. Approaching PD calmly and matter-of-factly will help them understand your condition as a natural event. The more accepting you are of your condition, the more children will be.

Use humor. Humor can often make difficult situations tolerable. Don't use humor to mask reality or hide your real feelings.

> *I owe a lot to my six beautiful daughters. They care for my every need. When they find something on Parkinson's in a publication, they send it to me. They call my doctor regularly and ask about new treatments. I don't know what I would do without them.*
>
> *Marie*
> *Age 68*

Children will know when humor isn't genuine. But when you can laugh at yourself and your condition, it makes the situation easier to handle.

Telling Your Employer

"Should I tell my employer?" is a question often asked by people newly diagnosed with PD. Perhaps a more accurate question is "When should I tell my employer?" Unfortunately, there is no clear-cut answer. Each person's situation is different. The kind of job you have will affect when you will need to tell your boss. For instance, an airline pilot or a brain surgeon with PD will likely have to tell his/her employer sooner than someone who sells insurance. How rapidly your disease progresses and how well your symptoms can be controlled with medications will also affect when you tell your employer. Also, the kind of relationship you have with your supervisor and the organization may affect how and when you inform them.

You can't predict the outcome of informing your employer. Your supervisor may make it easy for you to attend doctor's appointments and make accommodations in your work environment to make your job easier. Other times employers are less empathetic. You may be reassigned to other job duties or be pressured into early retirement. Remember, PD is a disability. You are protected under federal law from unlawful firing on account of it. However, it may prove difficult and costly to win such a case in court. Here are some guidelines to consider before talking with your employer:

- Discuss your work situation and any limitations you have at the workplace openly with your doctors.

- Ask your doctors about accommodations that might make it possible for you to continue being productive in your job.
- Make a list of the pros and cons of telling your employer. Realistically look at your situation and ask yourself, "Can I still do this job and do it well?"
- Have some suggestions for accommodation to offer your employer. Perhaps, like many telecommuters today, you can work out of your home.

Adapting to Changing Roles and Finding Focus

PD will invariably change your roles both at home and at work. It will likely change how you view yourself, too. It's important to keep in mind that you are not your disease. You happen to be a person with PD. Your condition is simply a part of who you are.

At home you may no longer be able to perform your usual tasks. This may affect how you feel about yourself. You may find your partner and children taking on responsibilities such as driving, paying bills, making decisions, and planning the social calendar that you used to do yourself or together.

In our household, our roles were changing. Since my handwriting was so poor, my wife now had to prepare the bills. I took over much of the shopping and cooking. While I didn't mind these changes in roles, I must say they took some getting used to.

For some people, nothing represents independence like the automobile. However, the changes in motor and concentration skills make it important for people with PD to be realistic about their ability to continue driving. Some willingly give up their driver's licenses. Others are less willing, cherishing their independence. At some point, it will be important to have your driving skills assessed by a professional driving instructor to determine whether it is still safe for you to drive.

Thus far I have mostly discussed coping with losses. But what are you going to put in place of those losses? It's vitally important that you reprioritize, finding new focus and meaning in your life.

For many of us, work defines who we are. We don't say, "I'm a loving, loyal person." Instead we say, "I'm a doctor (or lawyer, secretary, teacher, writer)." When that work role changes or disappears, we may find ourselves at a loss.

Not everyone with PD has to give up his/her job. Many individuals can still work effectively. If you have work you can still perform, stay with it as long as possible. If changes in your physical and mental capabilities make it difficult to do your job, look for ways to change your job or make accommodations that might enable you to keep working. With computers, faxes, cell phones, and other technological advances, perhaps you can work out of your home. If your current job becomes too difficult, consider another vocation. Take a look at your past experience and skills. How can you put those to work in another capacity?

When I feel overcome with anger and frustration I find something to laugh at in cartoons or on television. I am determined to remain independent for as long as possible. (I was also born with cerebral palsy.) PD has disrupted my teaching career, but I have made up my mind to deal with it in a positive way.

Kathleen
Age 60

Perhaps you could be a consultant or start your own business. Maybe you could find a less demanding job part-time. The point is to stay productive, to contribute for as long as you are able.

As time passed, I found myself becoming more and more restless. I felt I was wasting my life and contributing very little. Because I had been so busy in my medical practice, I had never developed hobbies. I knew I had better find a purpose and find it fast before I drove myself and my dear wife crazy. It occurred to me that I could use my knowledge and experience to write a book about medicine. As soon as I made the decision, I felt better. Once again, I was productive. I had set a realistic and challenging goal for myself. It felt great.

Patients experience a lot of setbacks. Those who have a means of coping, whether it be a sense of humor or a support system, really seem to persevere.
Alex, 46
Physician

Not everyone can or wants to continue working. Many people are near or at retirement age when they develop PD and would rather engage in other pursuits. That's fine, too, as long as those pursuits provide a sense of focus, purpose, fulfillment, and accomplishment. Becoming involved in church, community, or volunteer activities can shift focus from personal problems to helping others. Taking a class in an area of interest or teaching a class to adults or children can be very rewarding.

4

Your Doctor as Partner

With a chronic disease such as PD, a good relationship with your doctors is vitally important. After all, you and your doctors will likely deal with this disease together for many years to come. Many of us grew up believing that doctors are somehow magical, that their advice is always right, and that a patient's role is simply to do exactly as they instruct, no questions asked. Times have changed. The demands of a complicated and challenging disease such as PD require that you establish and maintain a strong partnership with your doctors. Each of you will bring information and expertise to the partnership. Your doctors and other professionals on your healthcare team will provide the medical and clinical expertise. You will bring expertise about yourself—how you feel both physically and emotionally and how those feelings change over time. As a partner in your healthcare, you have the right to question or reject any medication or surgical procedure. You also have the right to a second opinion. You and your doctors must cooperatively make decisions about your care. A strong partnership will help ensure that you get the best treatment for your condition.

Your Healthcare Team

People with PD usually have at least two doctors: a primary care physician and a neurologist. A *primary care physician* is your "regular" doctor, your family physician. He/she is the doctor you and your family have been seeing for some time. Usually a primary care physician is an internist, family physician, or general practitioner. In other words, he/she provides general medical care. Your primary care physician usually refers you to a specialist, the neurologist. Depending on your condition and your insurance plan, your primary care physician may follow and treat your disease, as well as any other health problems as they come up. Your insurance plan may allow you to see a neurologist or other specialist only periodically.

A *neurologist* is a doctor who has specialized training in disorders and treatment of the nervous system. Since PD is a nervous system disorder, it is important that you are evaluated by a neurologist. Ideally, your neurologist should make or confirm the diagnosis of PD, recommend symptomatic treatment, and monitor treatment.

I had six different doctors tell me I had Parkinson's disease before I finally believed it. Getting a second opinion is a good idea, but not to the extreme I did. Rather than wasting time denying it, take action immediately, especially when it comes to deciding which treatment option is right for you.

Curtis
Age 58

Just as many physicians have different interests and experience, so do neurologists. Within a specialty like neurology, some doctors continue their training in a specialized area now termed "movement disorders," that is, diseases that have movements as their symptoms. Some even go on to do clinical and research work in university-based PD research centers. If your community has one of these research centers, you will find qualified neurologists there. Wherever you live, look for a neurologist who has interest, training, and experience in treating patients with PD.

Depending on your symptoms, you may need other specialized treatment. For instance, some people with PD experience mental disturbances—difficult thoughts, feelings, and behaviors as well as losses in memory. A *psychiatrist*, a medical doctor with special training in mental health, can diagnose and treat mental disorders. He/she may use psychotherapy, marital and family counseling, and medications to help with PD-related mental health issues. A psychiatrist may see you initially and then refer you to another mental health provider like a *clinical psychologist* or a *social worker* for longer-term treatment. Often families with loved ones who have PD have a whole range of needs, including financial, emotional, and social. A social worker is not only trained in family and marital therapy but also can help you access other community services. (Such providers are often less expensive than psychiatrists. Who you see may depend on your health-insurance policy.)

If you have problems with self-care, employment, or leisure activities, your doctor may refer you to an *occupational therapist*.

> *I've learned how to be assertive in getting the information I need as a patient, whether its through literature or directly from a physician. It's especially important to ask questions if you don't understand the jargon healthcare professionals use.*
>
> *Leona*
> *Age 71*

He/she can help you choose adaptation equipment that will help you safely cope with many of your symptoms and make life easier.

A *physical therapist* can help you deal with mobility, posture, and balance problems. He/she is trained to assess such physical problems and prescribe appropriate exercises. In addition, a physical therapist can help you determine which leisure physical activities are best for you.

A *speech therapist* helps people improve communication and cope with swallowing difficulties.

A *massage therapist* can provide short-term help for stiff muscles and rigidity. Often health plans do not cover such services. Check your policy first.

If you need help with dietary matters, a *dietitian* can help. He/she can help you plan a healthy diet and devise ways to prepare meals that accommodate your limitations.

It's too easy to overlook your pharmacist as part of your healthcare. A pharmacist can do more than just dispense medications. He/she can answer your questions about medications, keep track of potentially dangerous drug interactions, and advise you on supplements and over-the-counter medications. The best strategy is to use only one pharmacy, preferably one that has a computer system for tracking all the drugs you're taking. Also, select a pharmacist who will take the time to carefully explain your medications and answer your questions.

Choosing the Right Doctor/Healthcare Team

A first step in taking an active role in your healthcare is to choose the right doctor and other members of your healthcare team. With a long-term disease such as PD, it's especially important that you and your health-care team develop a special bond. It's important that you have the right "fit," that you can talk honestly and openly with your physician and other health-care team members. They must demonstrate the time, energy, personality, and expertise to provide you with the best care. You must be able to trust that the advice your health-care professionals give you is entirely in your best interest.

Where do you find the right doctor and other specialists who can help you with your condition? Unless your insurance company is very restrictive, you may seek referrals from:

- friends, relatives, coworkers, and acquaintances
- other doctors, nurses, and pharmacists
- PD support groups
- a national PD Foundation office
- area hospitals or medical schools
- state or county medical associations (ask for a list of board-certified neurologists)
- area PD research centers
- your insurance company's preferred-provider list

A Word about HMOs

With the introduction of health maintenance organizations (HMOs), choosing the right doctor has become a bit more complicated. HMOs have changed the way we select our healthcare providers. Under most HMO plans, you must first see a primary care doctor before you can be referred to a specialist such as a neurologist. Some plans allow such a referral only under special circumstances. You also have to select a provider from their list of preferred providers. If you choose a doctor not on the preferred-provider list, your insurance will likely not cover the cost unless it has been preapproved by the administrator of your plan.

However, even under HMO plans, you have choices. Ask friends and coworkers who have the same insurance plan who they recommend. If you go to one of the doctors on your HMO's list and don't like him/her, find another preferred provider. Just because you have a particular type of insurance doesn't mean that you have to see a doctor with whom you're not comfortable.

If your primary care doctor seems hesitant to refer you to a specialist, be assertive. Tell him or her it's time you saw a neurologist. Make sure the specialist is covered under your plan.

What makes a good doctor or other healthcare specialist? For some people, it's important that he/she be on time. For others, it's more important that the doctor or specialist be personable. Only you can decide what's most important for you in your healthcare team. Take a moment to review the list below. Then make your own list and use it to select your healthcare team.

A Checklist for Evaluating the Right Healthcare Team

___Are you comfortable with this doctor/specialist? Does his/her personality "fit" with yours?

___Do you feel you could openly discuss all your concerns and feelings with this healthcare provider, even sensitive or potentially embarrassing subjects such as sexual or emotional problems?

___Do you feel you could ask this healthcare provider even "silly" questions?

___Does this doctor/specialist listen well and answer all your questions in language you can understand?

___If you don't understand something, is he/she willing to take the time to translate complex medical problems and medical jargon? Is he/she willing to use visual aids to further your understanding?

___Does this healthcare provider welcome you and your partner (or other patient advocate) as active partners in your treatment?

___Does he/she allow enough time for you during office visits so that you don't feel rushed?

___Does he/she seem interested in you and your condition?

___Is this person empathetic, able to put him/herself in your shoes?

___Is he/she on time?

___Does this doctor/specialist have experience treating PD patients? Special training?

___Does this doctor/pharmacist thoroughly explain your medications—how they work, what they're supposed to do, when and how to take them, side effects to watch out for, and what to do if you miss a dose?

___Does your healthcare professional try to educate you about PD by referring you to pamphlets and books and by talking about it during your visits?

___Is he/she willing to talk with you about alternative or experimental treatments?

___Does this doctor/specialist explain self-help strategies, such as exercise and diet?

___Is this doctor willing to refer you to the proper specialists as needed?

___Is he/she available in emergencies?

___Is he/she available by phone?

___Does he/she return your phone calls promptly?

Communicating with Your Healthcare Team

Good communication is the key to a strong partnership with your doctor and other members of your healthcare team. When you are first diagnosed and as your disease progresses, you will have many questions. Below are a few questions you may consider asking your primary care provider or neurologist.

Communication is a two-way street. You will not only need to ask your doctor and other PD specialists questions, you will need to provide them with honest, straightforward information about your condition, your feelings, and your ability to stick with your treatment plan. Let them know.

- how well your medications are working.
- if you experience any side effects from the drugs.
- about any other problems you are having with your treatment plan.
- about strategies you have discovered that make taking your medications or other parts of your treatment plan more effective.
- about any new symptoms you may have experienced.
- if you are planning to travel overseas.

Getting the Most from Your Office Visits

You will want to get the most from every visit with your doctors. Why? PD progresses slowly, so you will likely see your doctors only periodically. During visits, your doctors will likely perform a physical exam and specific physical tests to check your progress. He/she will want to observe your walking and check your manual dexterity. Occasionally, he/she will conduct laboratory tests to monitor your medications. Here are some tips for getting the most from your office visits.

Prioritize your visits. Know what you want to accomplish before you go to the doctor. Perhaps you want the doctor to adjust your medication dosage or talk about ways to cope with new, troubling symptoms. Plan ahead. You will get more done.

Don't waste time. Keep in mind that your doctor sees many patients. He/she has only a limited amount of time to spend with you. This is especially true under many HMO plans. Your time is valuable, too. Don't waste time on unrelated conversations or chitchat.

Invite your patient-advocate. Ask your partner or a close family member, friend, or caregiver to accompany you to the doctor's office. This person may act as your patient-advocate, one who will help you ask questions, give additional information to the doctor, take notes, and act in your best interest. It is especially important to have a patient advocate if you feel shy or intimidated about talking with the doctor or asking questions. If you prefer, your patient advocate may even accompany you into the exam room and/or into the doctor's office after the exam.

> *I'm convinced it isn't the pills the doctor gives you, but the time he gives you. If the doctor doesn't have time to listen, then it's time to find a new doctor.*
>
> *Mel*
> *Age 50*

Take a list. Make a list of questions and concerns you have and take it with you into the exam room. You would be surprised how often patients forget important issues they want to discuss once they see the doctor. A list will keep you on track.

Take notes. It's difficult to remember everything the doctor says. Don't be afraid to make notes while the doctor is talking. Or ask your patient-advocate to take them for you. Or take a tape recorder and record your conversation.

Be honest. Your doctor can help only if he/she has complete and honest information about your condition, your symptoms, and your compliance with your treatment program. Sometimes it's difficult to talk about certain topics such as sexual dysfunction or your feelings, but the more candid you are, the better your doctor will be able to help.

Be informed. Learn as much as you can from reading, from talking with others about PD, and from talking with your doctor. Be prepared to ask your doctor about new procedures and medications for treating PD. You may wish to subscribe to any of several newsletters dedicated to keeping people with PD up-to-date about new developments in treatment and research. Such newsletters are available from PD foundations and organizations, listed in the resource section of this book.

Even though the tremors add a new challenge to my golf game, I still go to the golf course and take a whack at it. If I'm not up to par, I don't play, but I still enjoy riding in the golf cart and cheering on my buddies.

Clinton
Age 62

The Case for Patient-Advocates

If you asked most people, "Do you want or need a patient advocate?" most would likely say no. We're not used to asking for help, especially the kind of intimate help a patient-advocate provides. Most of us would probably feel embarrassed about having someone else with us in the exam room. We believe we can speak for ourselves. We can handle this alone.

Not so. As a patient, you are not in a good position to act as your own advocate. The nature of PD can make it difficult to make good decisions on your own. In addition, strong emotions and mood swings can make it harder to act in a rational, objective manner.

> *Even as a doctor, I'm not a good patient-advocate for myself. Often I'm too close to my disease and too emotional about it to be able to objectively discuss it. My wife, who lives with and observes my disease and my symptoms on a daily basis, is more analytical about it. She's the one who tells the doctor about subtle new symptoms that have developed since my last visit. She's the one who remembers to let the doctor know about an easily-forgotten side effect of some medication.*

A well-informed mate, family member, friend, or caregiver who knows your history, your needs, and your desires is in the best position to help you help yourself and get you the best treatment possible.

5

Treatment for Parkinson's Disease

Today science has given us a much better understanding of how the brain works, what happens with PD, and how to treat it. While it is important for people with PD to have faith and be upbeat, it is equally important that they not be taken in by false claims of "miracle cures." To date, there are no drugs, herbal remedies, injections, manipulations, machines, surgery, or other treatments that "cure" the disease. The best symptomatic treatment options include drug therapy, surgery, and physical therapy.

Drug Therapy

A variety of medications can provide dramatic relief from the symptoms of PD. The right drugs can often help recover many lost body functions, protect against further disability, and help those with PD maintain independence for many years. Accordingly, it's important that you know as much as possible about these drugs. There is no one-size-fits-all treatment for PD. Your treatment needs to be tailored to you. Just as people vary widely in PD symptoms, they also vary in their responses to drug treatment. Some people do very well with a particular drug. Others may not be able to take the drug at all, or find that the drug does little to alleviate their symptoms. It's important to work closely with your doctor, letting him/her know how you are reacting to and tolerating particular drugs and dosages. Together you can find the right combination of medications that works for you.

You will need to be patient. All of us want our symptoms "fixed" immediately. Unfortunately, that's not how many PD drugs work. New drugs are usually introduced in low dosages and gradually increased over time. Often when one first begins taking an antiparkinson medication, it causes side effects such as nausea. Over time, these side effects usually lessen or disappear altogether. Also, many PD drugs take several months to develop their full therapeutic effects. Stay in close communication with your doctor, especially when starting new drug regimens. Don't stop taking your medications or change your dosage without talking with your doctor first. Stopping many of these drugs needs to be done gradually to reduce the chance of side effects. If you're having severe side effects or adverse reactions, let your doctor know right away. Sometimes these reactions are caused by other drugs you are taking, so your drug regimen may simply need adjustment.

Even though my physical appearance has changed, my inner beauty shines strong when I help others. When I do volunteer work with the elderly, it makes me focus on their problems rather than my own.

Ruth
Age 72

Since PD is a progressive disease, you will likely take different drugs at different stages. In the early stages, doctors often begin treatment with one or more of the less powerful drugs. More powerful drugs are usually reserved for later stages of treatment. Despite all the drugs available, not all of your symptoms may be alleviated completely.

Levodopa: The Gold Standard of PD Therapy

A major breakthrough was made in the symptomatic treatment of PD with the discovery of the drug, levodopa or l-dopa, which is the treatment of choice today. Levodopa enters the brain and is converted to dopamine, the chemical lacking in people with PD. Dopamine itself cannot be absorbed directly. Scientists have found that dopamine alone can't cross the *blood-brain barrier*, an intricate network of fine blood vessels and cells that filter blood before it reaches the brain. However, levodopa is able to pass through the blood-brain barrier and enzymes there convert it into dopamine. Levodopa allows many people with PD to live relatively normal, active, and productive lives for many years.

For me the two most important functions are exercise and my medications. I try to use the lowest dose I can and even go without medication for short periods of time in an effort to help prolong the drug's usefulness.

Lee
Age 80

Levodopa is combined with a second drug, *carbidopa,* which inhibits an enzyme that can destroy large amounts of levodopa before it reaches the brain. Consequently, more levodopa gets to the brain. Moreover, carbidopa also helps reduce side effects such as nausea, vomiting, abdominal distress, and heart problems.

If you or someone close to you has PD, you are probably familiar with the drug Sinemet, the brand name for carbidopa/

levodopa. This drug also comes in a slow-release form, Sinemet CR. The slow-release variety requires fewer repeat doses.

Sinemet is usually started in small doses. Then, over time, a doctor adjusts the dosage until the best clinical response is achieved and symptoms are controlled as best they can be. Even after a therapeutic dose is reached, it may take as long as two to three months to receive carbidopa/levodopa's full benefit. Over time, most individuals will need to have other drugs added to the Sinemet regimen. For the drug to remain effective as long as possible, doctors try to keep the levodopa dose as low as possible while still keeping symptoms in check.

While at least three-quarters of people with PD can be helped with carbidopa/levodopa therapy, it doesn't work equally well in treating all PD symptoms. Carbidopa/levodopa works well for bradykinesia and rigidity. However, it often only slightly improves tremors and may not help balance or other motor symptoms at all.

A troublesome problem for many people on carbidopa/levodopa therapy is the wearing-off effect. The drug loses its effectiveness. Consequently, pronounced PD symptoms begin to recur before the next scheduled dose. One can usually tell when the medication is wearing off: slowness and other motor symptoms recur. Sometimes symptoms may continue to worsen even after the next dose, which leads many people to believe the drug is responsible. It's not. The symptoms are likely caused from a combination

> *As the wife of a Parkinsonian it is very important to attend all doctors' appointments with my husband. When the doctor asks my husband questions, he seems to go blank or takes a long time to answer. I keep a written record of the visits. I like his doctor.*
>
> *Grace*
> *Age 72*

of disease progression and the long time it takes for the drug to be absorbed by the brain.

As PD progresses and levodopa is used over a long period of time, about 30 percent of PD patients experience on-off attacks, in which they "freeze," becoming immobile. Experts believe this occurs because over time more of the dopamine receptors in the brain disappear and/or lose their ability to take in the dopamine delivered by the levodopa. The freezing episodes may occur several times a day, lasting from a few seconds to a few minutes. These incidents often occur when attempting to enter a doorway or turn around. You may be able to devise some "tricks" which can help—such as attempting to march rather than walk. Still, at first, these attacks can be frightening so try to stay calm and wait for the storm to pass. Your physician may adjust dosages of your medications to help control these symptoms.

Freezing is a big problem for me. I heard about a new cane that has a lever that drops down on a patient's foot to help get him walking again. Investing in these tools is an investment in yourself.
Clyde
Age 70

Another problem resulting from the long-term use of levodopa is dyskinesia—involuntary nodding, jerking, or twitching which may be fast or slow, mild or severe. Controlling this disturbing symptom, when severe, can be difficult; again, it requires patience, knowledge and often the skill of a neurologist who can find the right balance of medications.

Potential Side Effects of Carbidopa/Levodopa

- nausea
- vomiting
- low blood pressure (orthostatic hypotension)

- heart arrhythmias
- involuntary movements—nodding, jerking, twitching (dyskinesia)
- restlessness
- mental changes
- dizziness

Getting the Most from Carbidopa/Levodopa

After ten years of coping with PD, I have learned the importance of taking my medications exactly as they are prescribed, especially taking them on time. I recall once not taking an extra dose with me when I left the house. I was almost paralyzed by the time I got home. It's a good thing I was not driving.

Take medications exactly on time. You need to follow a strict time schedule to prevent or reduce "off" times, when the drug isn't working.

Keep a dose with you. Carry your dose pack with you at all times. If you get stuck in traffic or are otherwise delayed for some reason, you'll still be able to take your dose on time.

Develop a reminder system. As we noted earlier, calendars, check-off lists, and alarms can help remind you when to take your medication. Some dose packs have alarms that can be set to go off at the right time. Ask your doctor about chewing tablets if you've missed a dose by an hour or less. It may give you faster relief.

Don't try to make up for missed doses. If you've missed a dose by a few hours, don't double your dosage to try and make up. It will only increase side effects. Take your regular dosage and get back on schedule.

For maximum absorption, take Sinemet sixty minutes before or after meals. Food in the stomach slows absorption and prevents the maximum amount of levodopa from getting to the brain.

Overcome nausea. If nausea is a problem, especially in the morning, try eating a few crackers or drinking a glass of juice with your dose.

Talk to your physician about low protein meals. A special low-protein diet has been developed for people taking levodopa since protein may interfere with the absorption of the drug. Levodopa rapidly disappears into the blood within 60 to 90 minutes. Anything that delays the drug getting into the bloodstream will also decrease the amount of the drug that reaches the brain. Levodopa is a type of amino acid that must attach itself to carrier molecules in the walls of the intestines to get into the blood. The bloodstream can only transport a certain number of these amino acids at a time. The more protein you eat, the more amino acids will be circulating in the blood, slowing the absorption of levodopa. Also, some researchers believe the wearing-off and on-off effects of PD therapy may be caused or worsened by too much protein in the diet. However, protein is required for our diets, so moderating may be better than lowering the amount used.

> *Since I was diagnosed with PD three years ago, my husband and I have relocated to be nearer a member of our family. Being near our daughter and her husband has been wonderful. I am fortunate that my medications have restored my energy levels.*
> LaVerne
> Age 73

Dopamine Agonists

These drugs attach to dopamine receptor sites in the brain, thereby mimicking the effects of dopamine. Consequently, a patient experiences relief from PD symptoms. Dopamine agonists may be used alone or in combination with levodopa. They often prompt a reduction in the dosage of levodopa 5 to 30 percent. Though generally not as effective as levodopa, dopamine agonists may be particularly helpful during the early stages of PD. Used in this way, they may equal the effectiveness of levodopa for the first one to three years of use. Dopamine agonists may also help patients who experience wearing-off or on-off problems with levodopa.

Commonly prescribed dopamine agonists include: bromocriptine (Parlodel), pergolide (Permax), pramipexole (Mirapex), and ropinirole (Requip).

Advantages of Dopamine Agonists

- may be used alone
- may reduce or eliminate many side effects of levodopa
- reduce the dosage of levodopa needed
- help calm nighttime leg cramping
- useful at any stage of the disease
- may help control tremors, rigidity, and slow movements
- may be taken with meals
- have a long half-life (It takes up to seven hours or more for half of a dosage to be used up.)

Despite the many advantages of dopamine agonists, their effectiveness is limited. They are not effective in treating postural problems, freezing, or dementia. Dopamine agonists have potential side effects, although not all of them have the same side effects.

Potential Side Effects of Dopamine Agonists

- nausea
- vomiting
- dizziness on rising (orthostatic hypotension)
- reduced appetite
- reddish discoloration of the skin
- stuffy nose (gradually disappears)
- confusion
- hallucinations
- increased dyskinesia
- scar-like tissue in the lining of lungs, gut, and deep abdominal tissue (rare)

We rarely think about the side effects of drugs. That is, until they affect us. I was taking the dopamine agonist bromocriptine and developed fibrosis, the scar-like tissue that can form in the lungs, in the gut, and in the deepest abdominal tissue. This rare complication occurs mostly in men over age sixty who have been taking forty milligrams or more of the drug for two years or longer. It's an insidious side effect that can cause major damage before it's discovered. Fortunately, my doctors discovered the fibrosis before the scarring irreparably damaged my lungs and gut. Gradually, they discontinued the bromocriptine. It takes about two years for the scar-like tissue to regress and repair itself. Note: this rare side effect occurs only with the agonists pergolide and bromocriptine. It has not been observed with the newer drugs Requip and Mirapex.

Anticholinergics

For many years, *anticholinergics* were the primary drugs used to treat PD. These drugs reduce tremors by blocking the action of *acetylcholine*, a neurotransmitter in the brain that influences motor functions. Sold under such brand names as Artane, Akineton, Cogentin, and Kemadrin, anticholinergics may also help prevent excessive sweating and drooling.

However, not everyone may be helped by anticholinergics. Experts say only about half of those prescribed anticholinergics respond. Many only respond for a short period of time, and most report only about 30 percent improvement. The drugs may be prescribed for mild to moderate symptoms but are usually ineffective in later stages of PD. The therapeutic dosages prescribed depend on which anticholinergic is used and on the individual's response to the drug. These drugs are not usually prescribed for older patients since they commonly cause psychiatric side effects such as confusion.

There is a lot of great information on the Internet, but you must always ask yourself if the source providing this information is reliable. Health organizations, universities and physicians are good sources of information.

Evelyn
Age 47

Potential Side Effects of Anticholinergics

- dry mouth
- dry eyes
- blurred vision
- memory loss, confusion, hallucinations
- difficulty urinating
- constipation
- increased heart rate (more common among the elderly)
- may worsen glaucoma unless counteracted with eye drops

Amantadine (Symmetrel)

Amantadine is an anti-viral medication used in the treatment of influenza. The antiparkingson's effects of this drug were discovered by accident when it was used to treat the flu in people who happened to have PD. Amantadine has been found to decrease involuntary movements (dyskinesia) in some late-stage PD patients. Scientists aren't sure how it works. It's believed that it may stimulate dopamine receptors in the brain.

Amantadine is sometimes used in the early stages of PD. More recently, scientists have found that this drug can decrease dyskinesias when used in late-stage PD. The drug may be used alone or in combination with other antiparkinson drugs such as anticholinergics or levodopa.

Potential Side Effects of Amantadine

- mottled skin (livido reticularis)
- swelling (edema)
- confusion
- blurred vision
- depression
- nightmares

When this drug loses its efficacy, it can ge stopped for a time, and may be effective when started again.

Enzyme Inhibitors

Enzyme inhibitors block the conversion of one substance into another. In the case of PD medications, the inhibitor of dopa decarboxylase blocks the action of an enzyme that breaks down levodopa. This action allows more levodopa to enter the brain and be converted to dopamine.

Selegiline (Eldepryl)

This inhibitor blocks the activity of an enzyme (*monoamine oxidase, type B*) that breaks down levodopa, allowing the levodopa to remain longer in the brain. Selegiline may be used during any stage of PD. Taken early in the disease, selegiline may improve symptoms and help delay the need to take levodopa for several months. The drug may also be used with levodopa to smooth out motor functions and to prolong "on" time. Some researchers suggest selegiline may provide some protection for neurons and may actually slow the progression of the disease.

However, selegiline is not without problems. Some doctors question the long-term safety of selegiline. Others believe because of its neuroprotective effect, it should be used by all people newly diagnosed with PD. Still others consider it a useful drug, especially when used in combination with other antiparkinson drugs. Animal studies suggest that selegiline may prolong life. Other studies suggest it may shorten the life span of people with PD. Further studies are needed to resolve this controversy. If you are taking selegiline, you may want to talk with your doctor about the pros and cons of continuing its use. The drug should only be taken before noon due to its metabolic breakdown into amphetamine which may preclude sleep if taken later.

Adverse drug interactions may occur when taking certain drugs with the enzyme inhibitor selegiline (Eldepryl, Deprenyl). According to the manufacturer and the FDA, the drugs listed below, which include popular antidepressants, should not be taken if you're on selegiline. However, some physicians report they prescribe low doses of antidepressants and find adverse interactions are rare. Still, talk to your physician about using any of the following:

- fluoxetine (Prozac)
- sertraline (Zoloft)
- paroxetine (Paxil)
- meperidine (Demerol)

Clearly, the painkiller, Demerol, is to be avoided. If taken, interactions such as fever, tremor, rigidity, and even death, may occur. Consider wearing a Medic-Alert bracelet to avoid dangerous drug interactions in case of an emergency.

Tolcapone (Tasmar)

One of the newer enzyme inhibitors for the treatment of PD, Tasmar has been shown to inhibit the enzyme COMT and peripheral breakdown of leodopa, allowing more of it to reach the brain over a longer period of time. It has also been shown to help the response to the drug Sinemet, making the transition from "on" and "off" periods smoother. It may take several months to realize the full benefit of Tasmar.

Advantages of Tasmar

- results in a smooth response to Sinemet
- decreases "wearing off" periods
- prolongs the duration of the action of dopamine
- works quickly—rapid onset
- allows up to a 25 percent reduction in the dosage of levodopa
- prolongs blood and brain levels of levodopa
- reduces the levels of potentially damaging free radicals
- allows a reduction in the dosage of dopamine agonists in combination therapy

- improves balance and motor activities
- acts as a stimulant and reduces feelings of fatigue

Potential Side Effects of Tasmar

- diarrhea (This side effect is usually delayed for four to six months. It rarely appears after the first six months.)
- dizziness on rising (postural hypotension)
- difficulty sleeping
- vivid dreaming

Tasmar Warning

The manufacturer of Tasmar reports that three people out of 60,000 taking the drug died of liver failure. These individuals were taking 200 milligrams of the drug three times a day. Accordingly, the Food and Drug Administration (FDA) has recommended that Tasmar be reserved only for severe cases of PD that are not helped by other therapies. If your doctor allows you to continue taking the drug, you will need to sign a release form and have laboratory liver-function tests frequently. Be sure to talk with your doctor before stopping Tasmar. Abruptly stopping the drug may cause a rebound of PD symptoms or other significant side effects.

Drugs That May Interfere with PD Medications

Some drugs prescribed for conditions other than PD may adversely affect dopamine in the brain. Such drugs may reduce the effectiveness of PD drugs. If a doctor prescribes any of the drugs listed below, be sure the doctor knows you have PD and is aware that the drug may alter your symptoms.

Antidepressants

> phenelzine (Nardil)
> tranylcypromine (Parnate)
> fluoxetine (Prozac)
> sertraline (Zoloft)

Antiepileptic Drugs

> phenytoin sodium (Dilantin)

Antipsychotic Drugs

> haloperidol (Haldol)
> lithium (Lithobid)
> chlorpromazine (Thorazine)
> trifluoperazine (Stelazine)
> fluphenazine (Trilafon)
> thioridazine (Mellaril)

Antinausea Drugs (Can compete with dopamine)

> prochlorperazine (Compazine)
> metoclopramide (Reglan)

Blood Pressure Drugs (Can block dopamine receptors)

> reserpine (Serpasil)
> alpha-methyldopa (Aldomet)
> rauwolfia serpentina (Raudixin)

Using Medications Safely and Effectively

To treat the symptoms of PD, you may need to take a number of medications. Many PD drugs must be taken precisely—the right dose at exactly the right time. With so many medications to keep track of, it is important that you develop an easy-to-use system that simplifies drug taking and helps you remain as independent as possible. Here are some tips:

Use a medication chart. Ask your doctor or pharmacist to provide a medication chart to keep track of your prescription and over-the-counter medications. Or make your own. On a piece of paper make several categories: brand and generic names of the medication, your dosage, what the drug looks like, when to take it, and any special instructions.

Use a daily or weekly pill organizer. Available at pharmacies, plastic pill boxes allow you to count out each day's pills. An egg carton works great, too.

Remind yourself when to take your medications. As noted earlier, there are any number of ways to help yourself remember to take your medications on time. Set your watch or alarm clock. Put the drugs where you will see them. For instance, if you take drugs first thing in the morning, put them in the bathroom by your toothbrush or in the kitchen where you eat breakfast.

Have one doctor oversee your medications. If you have multiple health problems and/or more than one doctor, the chance increases for dangerous drug interactions. Ask your primary healthcare provider or your neurologist to oversee all your medications. Have him/her review all the medications you're currently taking, including any over-the-counter medications, vitamins, minerals, and herbal supplements. Also, be sure all your doctors exchange case notes with each other.

Take all your drugs with you to the hospital and/or emergency room and to the doctor's office. Doctors need to know exactly what you're taking.

Choose one pharmacy. Find a pharmacist who will keep track of all your drugs and watch for dangerous drug interactions.

Many pharmacies are now computerized, which makes drug tracking easy.

Don't change your dosage or stop taking medications without first talking to your doctor.

Let your doctor know about adverse side effects. Don't wait for your next appointment. Call your doctor and let him/her know right away. Perhaps the drug or dosage can be changed.

Ask your pharmacist to clearly mark the outside of each drug container with instructions.

Keep medications in their original containers to avoid dangerous mix-ups.

Never use someone else's drugs.

Never use old or outdated drugs. They may have lost their potency.

Use a pill cutter. If your prescription requires you take half-pills, pill cutters that will give you an exact cut are available at pharmacies. Also, placing the pills in a freezer for an hour or so will allow you to cut them without crumbling. If cutting the pills is too difficult or exacting a task for you, ask someone else to do it.

Ask to have your pills blister packed. This will allow you to see exactly what pills you should take each day.

Keep extra doses with you. Pack a few doses of medication, a can of juice, and a few crackers in your car, office, and places you visit frequently. Or keep a fanny pack loaded with your prescriptions and juice to give you more freedom. You won't have to return home just to take medications on time.

Store medications in a locked cupboard away from children.

Learn about Your Medications

It is your responsibility to learn about the drugs you're taking. Ask your doctors these questions about each drug prescribed for PD and other health problems you might have:

- What are the generic and brand names of this drug?
- Is there a cheaper, generic form of this drug available that works equally well?
- What is this drug intended to do?
- How often and how long should I take this drug?
- How will this drug interact with other drugs? Are there any drug combinations I should avoid?
- Should I take this drug with food or on an empty stomach? Should I avoid any foods when taking this drug? May I use alcohol with this drug?
- How long will it take for this drug to work?
- What side effects should I expect?
- What dangerous side effects or adverse reactions should I watch out for? What should I do if I have such a reaction?
- What should I do if I miss a dose?
- How should I store this drug?

Also ask your pharmacist to give you patient information sheets, written information about side effects, instructions about when to call your doctors, dosage directions, a listing of conditions that indicates when the drug should not be taken, and any other special instructions.

A Word about Taking Drugs for Life

Many people find difficult the idea of taking drugs for the rest of their lives. They may say, "I've never taken a pill in my life." They may pride themselves on "being natural," taking few if any drugs or other chemicals. Some people are so adamant about not taking drugs, they try to treat PD the "natural way" with various herbs and concoctions from health-food stores, rigorous diets, and vitamin and mineral supplements. Unfortunately, none of these strategies appear to have an effect on PD symptoms. It's like a person trying to control diabetes without insulin. There is no evidence that any other remedy works as well as the chemical replacement therapy achieved with PD medications combined with sensible self-help. At least for now, effectively treating PD means taking medications for the rest of your life.

Praying comforts me. I have faith that God will give me the strength to conquer my weaknesses.

Verna
Age 78

The good news is that new classes of drugs are being developed all the time to treat PD symptoms. Unlike older drugs, the new drugs not only relieve symptoms but may also protect neurons in the brain. These new drugs may be capable of actually slowing the progression of the disease, reducing the need for powerful drugs with adverse side effects and improving the quality of life for people with PD.

Surgical Treatments

Neurosurgery to treat PD symptoms was first performed in the 1930s. Surgery usually involves damaging specific areas of the brain involved in motor functions in an attempt to reduce severe symptoms such as an uncontrollable tremor. Since the discovery of antiparkinson drugs, especially l-dopa, surgery has become much less common. However, not everyone can take L-dopa or other antiparkinson drugs. Others may still suffer severe tremors and other symptoms despite drug treatment. Recently, a number of doctors have rekindled interest in brain surgery for PD.

NOTE: If you should consider one of these surgeries, it is imperative that you thoroughly investigate the credentials of the surgeon. These surgical procedures should be done only by experienced neurosurgeons who use micro-electronic recording equipment which can pinpoint the exact area of the brain affected.

There are four types of surgical procedures for PD:
- Pallidotomy
- Thalamotomy
- Electrical Stimulation
- Neural Implants

Pallidotomy

First introduced in the 1940s, *pallidotomy* involves inserting a probe in the brain and destroying a part of the brain tissue called the *globus pallidus*, which is involved in the transmission of brain signals for movement. When pallidotomy works, it can reduce or eliminate tremors, slowness of movement, abnormal movements, stiffness, balance difficulties and freezing, and improve gait. In some patients, successful pallidotomy allows them to take less l-dopa or to take it with better results.

If you want to be the very best you can be you have to accept who you are. Take what you have, nourish it and watch yourself blossom.

Pauleen
Age 61

During pallidotomy, a halo frame is placed over the head of a patient. A picture of the brain is taken by MRI or CAT scan (*computerized axial tomography*). The patient is awake under local anesthesia to enable him/her to describe sensations as the surgery progresses. A larger metal frame, or *stereotactic frame*, is placed over the halo frame to guide the insertion of a probe deep into the globus pallidus, and the surgeon drills a small hole in the skull. Once the probe is in the proper position, the doctor applies an electrical current through the probe into the pallidum, lesioning it. If the surgery works as planned, the patient's abnormal movements disappear immediately. Often, the tremors as well as the slowness and rigidity subside. Unfortunately, because the current procedure is only a few years old, doctors don't know much about the long-term effects of pallidotomy.

Some surgeons believe that the globus pallidus should be lesioned on both sides of the brain for best results. Others contend the procedure should be performed only on one side. It's clear that bilateral procedures carry greater risk. At this time, most authorities do not recommend the two-sided procedure.

Until I underwent a pallidotomy by an experienced surgeon, I was nearly a total invalid with frequent episodes of freezing and severe dyskinesia. Since the surgery, I am now independent again and able to resume my daily activities. For me the results of the surgery were like a miracle.

Doug, 63
Retired M.D.

Although both pallidotomy (and thalamotomy) have been made safe and more effective with the use of new imaging techniques such as MRI and CAT scans and frames, the procedures still carry risks of potentially serious complications. Some of the side effects following surgery, however, are only temporary.

Potential Complications of Pallidotomy

- stroke caused by bleeding from damaged blood vessels
- confusion
- sleepiness
- weakness of facial muscles
- weakness of arm and leg muscles
- speech difficulties

- problems swallowing
- personality changes
- problems concentrating
- increase in appetite and weight gain
- visual problems, including loss of half of vision, and (rarely) blindness
- balance problems when walking

Are You a Good Candidate for Pallidotomy?

You may be a candidate for pallidotomy if you are
- severely disabled and have failed to respond to all antiparkinson medications.
- unable to take antiparkinson medications, or if medications are ineffective or worsen symptoms.
- younger than seventy years.
- mentally competent.
- have a tremor, abnormal movements (dyskinesia), and motor fluctuations.
- in good general health.

Thalamotomy

Thalamotomy destroys a small portion of the *thalamus*, a message-relay station deep inside the brain. When done on one side of the brain, it often relieves severe tremors on the opposite side of the body. First introduced in the 1940s, thalamotomy gained favor because it reduced PD tremors more effectively than did pallidotomy. New surgical techniques have made the procedure safer; however, it is not without possible complications.

Potential Complications of Thalamotomy

- convulsions or seizures
- disturbances in gait and balance

- severe speech and swallowing difficulties, especially when done on both sides of the thalamus
- problems with memory
- bleeding into the brain (mortality less than one percent)

Are You a Good Candidate for Thalamotomy?

Keep in mind that about 60 percent of PD patients experience tremor; of this group, about 10 percent suffer from disabling tremor. Accordingly these individuals stand to gain the most from the surgery. This procedure may be an option for you if you are

- experiencing intractable tremor
- unable to carry out the activities of daily living
- disabled occupationally or socially
- not responding to PD medications

Electrical Stimulation

This procedure carries less risk than the surgical procedures since it does not involve destroying any brain tissue. Instead, a section of the brain is stimulated with high-frequency electrical charges. It is believed this stimulation paralyzes nerve cells that become overly active and send messages that cause tremors. It is, however, more costly than lesioning procedures. The symptomatic relief depends on the area of the brain stimulated. Stimulation to the thalamus controls tremor only. Stimulation to the globus pallidus treats balance and rigidity problems, but not tremor. Another procedure, which may be approved for future use, involves stimulating the subthalamic nucleus in the brain. This procedure is thought to work in a more central area that would help to relieve all symptoms of PD.

Patients choosing this form of treatment undergo two separate surgeries consecutively. In one operation, a small battery, about the size of a cigarette pack, is implanted in the shoulder, under the clavicle. The battery will last two to five years, at which time a new one must be inserted. In the second procedure, a wire probe is guided into the brain. The patient is awake during both surgeries in order to communicate with doctors as they determine if the stimulation is beginning to control symptoms.

Once the stimulator is implanted, the patient uses a hand-held magnet to turn the stimulator on and off at will. In most cases, the tremor stops within one to three seconds of stimulation. The tremor returns, however, after the stimulator is turned off. In order to lengthen battery life, most patients turn off their stimulators at night.

Potential Complications and Side Effects of Electrical Stimulation

- hemorrhage
- stroke
- infection
- abnormal movement, muscle contraction, visual flashes that can result from improper placement of electrode
- electrode breakage
- need for battery replacement

Are You a Good Candidate for Electrical Stimulation?

This procedure can be helpful if you
- are unable to take antiparkinson medications, or medications are ineffective for all symptoms.
- have a disabling tremor and have undergone one-sided (unilateral) thalamotomy.
- have a severe tremor and want to avoid permanent, invasive surgery.
- have undergone a unilateral pallidotomy and do not want to risk a bilateral procedure. (Bilateral stimulation of the globus pallidus is possible with electrical stimulation.)

Neural Implants

In the 1980s, neurosurgeons in Sweden and China tried transplanting bits of live brain tissue from aborted fetuses into the brains of PD patients. The idea was that if these cells "took hold," they might make the brain of a person with PD produce more dopamine. However, success with this procedure has been slow, and moral controversy gave rise to a long-standing ban on fetal-tissue research. The ban was lifted in 1993, making further exploration of this surgery possible. Still, there are plenty of unanswered questions, and the surgery is considered experimental. It will likely be ten or more years before neural implants produce any real hope for treatment.

Physical Therapy

PD may cause problems in posture, deformities of the legs and arms, and gait disturbances. A program of physical therapy tailored to the individual may help control these problems. You, your doctor, and your physical therapist should work together to develop a program that may include:

Active and passive exercises. Active exercises are movements that can help you improve your range of motion, coordination, and speed of movement. Passive exercises include various stretches and manipulation by a physical therapist to help relieve muscle rigidity and stiffness.

Gait training. This training may improve how you walk by helping you learn proper foot placement, arm swing, and how to be better balanced.

Daily-life activities. A physical therapist can help you develop techniques to make daily activities easier to accomplish.

Heat, ice, electrical stimulation, and hydrotherapy. Your physical therapist may use heat, cold, electricity, or water therapy to treat your symptoms.

Other Therapies

It is important to maintain as much coordination and manual dexterity as possible. *Occupational therapies,* including craft projects, can help. Look for activities that you enjoy and that are safe for your condition. If you develop speech difficulties, speech therapy can often help. Speech therapists can provide exercises and techniques to overcome problems such as nasal monotone and softness in the voice.

6

Helping Yourself with Exercise

Regular exercise is one of the most important self-help strategies for coping with PD. The phrase "use it or lose it" definitely applies when it comes to PD. That's not to say it's easy. Even healthy people have difficulty getting and staying fit. Most avoid exercise altogether or try a few sessions and quit. With PD, the fatigue, limited movement, stiffness in the muscles and joints, and sometimes even breathing difficulties make exercise even less appealing.

Research and the experiences of thousands of people with PD confirm that exercise is vitally important for maintaining optimum motor functions. A study conducted by doctors at Emory University School of Medicine in Atlanta, Georgia, finds that both stretching and aerobic exercise is helpful for those with PD. Study subjects walked or ran forty minutes per day three times a week for twelve weeks. Their cardiovascular fitness improved by more than 30 percent, their motor disability improved by 22 percent, and their movement time improved by 37 percent.

Exercise will not stop PD, but it may improve your body strength so that you are less disabled. It may also improve balance, help you overcome gait problems, strengthen particular muscles, and improve speech and swallowing. Exercise vigorous enough for you to work up at least a light sweat may also make you feel better emotionally and help lift depression. Exercise releases endorphins, the body's own "feel-good" chemicals. Perhaps most importantly, a regular exercise program may help you feel more in control and give you a sense of accomplishment. If you participate in a structured class or program, exercise may help keep you connected with others and feel less isolated.

Exercise may also help prevent muscle and joint injury commonly associated with PD. Each day we perform thousands of automatic movements with our bodies, continuously stretching our ligaments and muscles. When the automatic system of movement breaks down, one must consciously think out each movement before performing it. Loss of automatic movements may lead to stiffening of the muscles and ligaments. Over time, joints may lose their range of motion.

When a person with PD tries to perform movements that are beyond the limited range or capacity of the ligaments and muscles, injuries such as sprains or strains are likely to occur. Regular exercise may help prevent such problems.

Benefits of Exercise

A regular exercise program may help you
- increase muscle strength.
- improve balance.
- overcome gait problems.
- decrease speech/swallowing problems.
- improve mood and lift depression.
- reduce muscle and joint injuries.
- feel more in control.

- achieve a sense of accomplishment.
- reduce feelings of isolation.

I exercise every day. I'm convinced that daily exercise for the past ten years has kept me out of a wheelchair. While exercising gets a bit more difficult as each month passes, I don't intend to give up exercising until I absolutely have to—and that's going to be quite a while from now.

Exercise That Works for You

Many PD patients make a program of regular aerobic, stretching, and strengthening exercises a priority in their treatment plan. Here are some tips for an effective and safe exercise program. Seek the approval of your physician before doing any of the exercises listed here.

Begin slowly. Muscles and joints unaccustomed to physical activity respond slowly. Start slowly and increase activity gradually over time. Trying to do too much too soon will only result in sore muscles and possible injury.

Choose an exercise regimen that you can easily fit into your daily routine. It doesn't do any good if you choose an exercise plan that you don't have the time, place, or physical capacity to perform. Choose one that you can and will do consistently. Also, choose one that you like. You will more likely stick with it.

If it hurts, stop. Don't push yourself to the point of pain. Slight discomfort is okay, but pain is a definite signal to stop what you're doing. If exercise consistently causes pain, talk with your doctor and/or physical therapist.

Lift your toes. Bring your toes up with every step you take. You will have less tendency to trip or misstep. Also use toe lifting to "unglue" your feet and legs, relieve muscle spasm, and reduce the possibility of a fall.

Create a wide base. When standing, walking, or turning, spread your legs wide (about twelve inches) to provide a wider base and help prevent falling.

Turn with small steps. Practice turning with a wide stance and small steps at least fifteen minutes every day until it becomes your natural style.

Look up. When walking, it is common for people with PD to stoop and watch their feet. Try to straighten up and look straight ahead.

Practice proper walking. When walking, use large steps. Your toes should rise up. As you step forward your heels should hit the ground. Practice walking sideways, backwards, and in circles several times a day.

Practice rapid movements. To improve your balance, move rapidly forward, backward, right, and left for five minutes at a time several times a day.

Overcome gravity. If getting out of a chair or bed is a problem, practice rising very quickly to overcome inertia and the pull of gravity. Be sure both feet are planted firmly beneath your chair or bed. Practice ten to twenty times a day. Put three- or four-inch blocks under the back legs of your favorite chair to make getting up easier. Chairs that propel you could be dangerous; check with your neurologist before buying these.

Swing your arms. When you walk, practice swinging your arms freely. This takes the weight off your legs, lessens fatigue,

> *Sometimes family and friends treat me as though I am fragile. They tell me to take it easy and I tell myself to keep moving. They have good intentions, but I need to do what's best for me.*
>
> *William*
> *Age 70*

and loosens the arms and shoulders. As one arm swings forward, the other should swing back. As your right arm moves forward, swing your left leg forward.

Balance the list. Some people with PD find themselves listing to one side or another. Try carrying hand weights or a shopping bag loaded with books on the nonlisting side to balance the load and decrease your body's bend.

Consider an in-home exercise machine. Bad weather can make it easy to put off exercising. Consider buying a treadmill, stationary bike, or other in-home exercise machine if you are unable to work out elsewhere.

March to the music. Try using music to help you maintain a steady gait, especially if you're experiencing freezing problems. Music can also make your exercise more interesting and enjoyable.

Keep your legs strong. Be sure to include some exercises that improve your leg strength. Strong legs will enable you to remain active longer and help prevent falls.

Strengthen those abs. Strong stomach muscles are important, especially if you suffer from back pain. Make sure your exercise routine includes "crunches," modified sit-ups, or other abdominal-strengthening exercises.

Consider yoga. This ancient art has a number of gentle stretching and strengthening postures that you should find quite helpful. Even people who are bedridden can use some of the postures.

> *I have done miracles for myself with exercise. People who saw me with a walker can hardly believe it's me. As they say, if you don't use it, you'll lose it.*
>
> *Stephen*
> *Age 68*

Avoid rubber- or crepe-soled shoes. They can grip the floor and trip you up.

Practice, practice, practice. If any task proves difficult, such as buttoning a shirt or getting out of bed, practice it at least twenty times a day to improve performance.

A Word about Expectations

Your expectations should not be unrealistically high. When you were well, you may have worked out and quickly made noticeable gains in muscle strength and cardiovascular endurance. It will be different with PD. Don't be discouraged if your muscle strength and endurance show little or no improvement. Your disease is continuing to progress. Your exercise program is simply helping you to cope with the progression of symptoms, especially the more disabling ones. It's enough that the exercise is helping you maintain a better quality of life and giving you a sense of control and accomplishment.

Exercise has helped me feel stronger, less fatigued. Yoga postures in particular have improved my posture and balance. Walking relieves my nausea and improves my bowel and bladder function. However, exercise is not a cure-all. It hasn't improved activities such as writing, buttoning, or tying shoes, all of which require fine motor skills.

What Kind of Exercise Should You Do?

All kinds of exercises may help. Your choice depends on your symptoms, your age, your physical strength, and your interests. The best program is one that combines a number of activities and continually changes as your symptoms and capabilities change. Your doctor and/or physical therapist can help you develop a program that is right for you.

Daily-activities exercise. This is the work you do in day-to-day living—household chores, bathing, dressing, grooming, shopping and so on. While this type of exercise won't improve your aerobic endurance (fitness of your heart and lungs), it will help keep you limber.

Doctor-prescribed activities. Your doctor may prescribe special exercises to prevent problems from muscle stiffness, to protect affected parts of your body from getting worse, or to recover functions that you may have lost.

Preventive exercises. These exercises help prevent potential problems. Preventive walking exercises are especially helpful. For instance, walking with a deliberately wide gait and small steps with your eyes looking straight ahead is a good exercise to help straighten posture, improve gait, and prevent falling.

Corrective exercises. Repetitively practice these exercises to help prevent movement limitations at particular joints. Getting out of a chair rapidly over and over will improve limitations in movements of the hip and leg joints due to tightened or shortened muscles.

Recreational exercises. These are fun activities like golf, dancing, bowling, swimming, hiking, or other activities that fit your interests. Recreation may not only help keep your muscles and joints flexible and strong but also help you interact with others.

Dr. Cram's Exercise Routine

I have developed this exercise program for myself. It combines stretching exercises to keep my joints and muscles limber with strengthening exercises. Many of these exercises are adaptations of yoga postures. Some or all of these exercises may work for you. Check with your doctor and/or physical therapist before trying them.

Proper Breathing. While exercising, always be sure to breathe out whenever doing the "work" part of an exercise. For instance, exhale when you stretch or lift a weight. Inhale as you relax. This will help prevent injuries, make the exercises easier to perform, and put you at ease.

Low Back Stretch. Lie flat on your back and bend your knees. Clasp your knees with your hands, pulling your legs toward your chest. You will feel a stretch in your lower back. Hold for a slow count of 10. Repeat this exercise as often as you like. It's a great way to loosen a stiff back in the morning.

Long Body Stretch. Lying flat on your back, raise your arms over your head and stretch your entire body as far as you can.

Shoulder Stretch. While standing, place both arms behind your back, clasping your fingers together. Straighten your arms and raise them as high as you are able. Hold them for at least a count of 10 or longer if you can. This is a great exercise for straightening your back.

> *Worrying seemed to make my muscle rigidity worse. Since I've been controlling my stress with deep breathing exercises, I feel less stiff and can think more clearly.*
>
> *Marla*
> *Age 62*

Hip Twist. Lie on the floor on your back. Bring your knees up into a slightly bent position. Now place one leg over the top of the opposite knee, allowing the upper leg to press down on the bottom leg. Keep your shoulders pressed to the floor. Let the bottom leg stretch only as far as it will comfortably go. You will feel a stretch in your lower back. Hold for a count of 20. Slowly bring your legs back to the flat lying position. Repeat with the opposite leg.

Neck Stretches. Lie on your back on the floor. Without using a pillow, rotate your head slowly back and forth from side to side. Do 15 to 20 rotations. Then raise your head up, alternately tilting your neck back and pulling your chin to your chest. Repeat 25 to 50 times. These exercises will increase the range of motion in your neck and reduce stiffness.

Single-Leg Strap Stretches. Sitting on the floor with both legs extended straight out in front of you, loop a strap or towel over one foot and bend the opposite knee out to the side. Using both hands to hold the strap, pull toward your body. You should feel stretching in your lower back and the back of your leg. Hold for a count of 15 to 20. Repeat on the opposite side.

Double-Leg Strap Stretches. Sitting on the floor with both legs extended straight out in front of you, loop a strap or towel over both feet. Grasping the strap or towel with both hands, pull toward your body, stretching and holding for a count of 15 to 20.

Side Stretches. Stand with a wide stance. Lift your left arm over your head, palm facing toward the midline of the body. Slowly bend at the waist on the right side, allowing the weight of your raised arm to help you stretch. You should feel a stretch on your left side. Hold for a slow count of 10. Repeat on the opposite side.

Waist Twist. Standing with a wide stance and hands on your hips, slowly twist your head and torso toward the right side as far as you can. Hold for a count of 10. Then twist back to the center and repeat on the opposite side.

Wall Squats. Stand about 8 inches from a wall. Facing the wall, bend your legs at the hips and knees, lowering yourself into a squatting position. Use the wall for support if needed. Hold this position for a slow count of 10. Then slowly rise up to a standing position. This exercise is difficult for many people. However, it may add to vitally needed leg strength.

Arm Weight-lifts. Lie on your back with hand weights (dumbbells) weighing 8 pounds or less in each hand. Hold the weights parallel to your body with your elbows tucked to your sides. Raise your arms until they are extended straight out. Hold briefly in the fully extended position, then slowly lower the weights to the starting position. Work up to 50 lifts. Then hold the weights near your shoulders at right angles to your body and lift them to the fully extended position. Hold briefly and lower. Work up to 50 lifts.

Foot-Grasp Back Stretch. Sit on the floor with your legs extended in front of you, flexed about 45 degrees. Bend your upper body as far as you can, extend your arms forward, and grasp the soles of your shoes with both hands. Pull forward toward your feet, gently stretching your lower back. Hold for 10 seconds, if possible. (Stop immediately if you feel pain.) Slowly work up to holding for at least 30

> *I have found exercising and staying very busy is the perfect way for me to combat PD. Swimming three days a week and working in my garden growing unusual flowers and plants does not leave time to fret.*
>
> *A.H.*
> *Age 70*

seconds. You will find this is great exercise for relieving lower back pain and taking the kinks out.

Partial Sit-ups with Weights. Lie flat on your back. With your knees bent and your arms at your sides, grasp a hand weight in each hand. Slowly raise your upper body off the floor and curl toward your knees, keeping the small of your back and your feet on the floor. Slowly curl back down to the resting position. Slowly work up to 50 sit-ups. This exercise strengthens abdominal muscles, important for preventing lower back pain.

> *I was concerned about my bent posture and always made a conscious effort to walk as straight as I could. Then a friend who is a yoga expert taught me some yoga stretches. After a few months of practicing the yoga postures, I not only felt better, my back had straightened considerably. I have added these yoga exercises to my daily routine as well as some light weights to work my upper body. My entire exercise program, which includes 30 to 45 minutes of walking outdoors or on a treadmill, takes just over an hour a day to complete. I try to do this program every day regardless of the weather or my location.*

A reminder: remember the importance of checking with your healthcare professional before beginning any exercise program.

7

Day-to-Day Coping

Coping with PD every day can be difficult. PD affects your whole life, from socializing with friends to earning a living. Everyday things you previously did with ease such as buttoning your shirt or rising from a chair can be a chore. PD requires you to learn a whole new way of living and coping, especially if you plan to remain as active as possible. This chapter is devoted to practical strategies and getting the assistance you need to help you better face the challenges of daily life.

Helping Yourself with Support

Many organizations like the National Parkinson Foundation and the Parkinson Disease Foundation (see Resources) sponsor support groups for people with PD and their loved ones. There are plenty of organizations to choose from: patient groups, patient/partner groups, caregiver groups, and groups for the entire family. Some PD support groups are targeted to specific ages like those for young-onset PD.

Many people, especially those newly diagnosed with PD, resist joining a support group. They believe they can face their disease alone. They don't want to be associated with "those sick people." For most, this initial resistance fades as they come to grips with their disease.

A support group can be a vital link in your self-help education network. It may help you and your loved ones

- understand more about PD and the physical limitations imposed by the disease.
- become aware of resources in the community such exercise programs, home healthcare services, and sources of adaptive equipment.
- obtain referrals to qualified healthcare professionals in your area who have experience with PD.
- talk about your fears and concerns in a supportive environment.
- develop ways to deal with feelings like anger, guilt, and helplessness.
- stay motivated to use exercise and other self-help strategies to maintain the best quality of life possible.
- communicate more effectively with your healthcare team.
- learn about the latest developments in PD research and treatment.
- find practical ways of coping with everyday challenges.

How do you find support groups? Start with your community's local chapter of the National Parkinson Foundation or the Parkinson Disease Foundation. If your community doesn't have a local chapter, call or write to the foundation's national headquarters (see Resources) and ask about forming a support group. You may also locate support groups through:

- your local hospital.

- your local hospital.
- your doctor.
- friends or associates who have PD or a similar neurological disorder.
- your community's mental health association.
- a PD research center in your area.

Helping Yourself with a Healthful Diet

Eating a well-balanced diet is important for everyone's good health. It is especially important for people with a chronic disease such as PD. However, there is no specific diet, vitamin, mineral, or herbal supplement that can cure PD or slow the progression of the disease. That's not to say you can't help yourself with a good diet.

There are plenty of dietary issues for someone with PD. Swallowing may be difficult or slow. PD slows the speed at which food moves through the digestive tract. It takes longer for the stomach to empty. With the slowing of digestion, constipation may become a problem. Some people with PD experience decreased appetite, changes in smell, and nausea (from antiparkinson medications), all of which may make eating less enjoyable and cause weight loss. A poor diet may interfere with the absorption of antiparkinson drugs like levodopa. Careful food planning in consultation with a dietitian may help you prevent many diet-related problems.

Generally speaking, people with PD require the same nutrients recommended for healthy people. Many of the same principles of good eating apply. A few additional dietary principles are especially helpful for people with PD.

Eat a variety of foods every day. Include vegetables, fruits, breads, pasta, rice, grains, eggs, meat, poultry, and fish.

Eat less fat. High-fat diets have been linked to heart disease. Be especially aware of foods loaded with saturated fat and cholesterol, such as fatty red meats. You can lower the fat in your diet by eating more fish, skinless poultry, and other lean meats. Eat less butter, oil, cheese, and ice cream. Drink low-fat milk. Substitute other lower-fat dairy products for higher-fat ones. If you need to add calories to your diet, try adding complex carbohydrates rather than fats.

Eat more complex carbohydrates. Starches, breads, and cereals—especially those rich in fiber—are not only a good source of energy, vitamins, and minerals but may also help you stay regular.

Maintain a healthy weight. Mobility is more difficult with excess weight. Get to and maintain a healthy weight. Weigh yourself weekly. Weight loss may be a sign of poor nutrition. If weight loss is a problem, talk with your doctor or dietitian about a liquid supplement.

Eat small meals frequently. Since your digestion is slowed with PD, eating smaller meals will help your body better digest and utilize foods.

Take a multivitamin. Most people get plenty of vitamins and minerals with a balanced diet. However, most people with chronic illnesses like PD have enough nutritional risks that it doesn't hurt to take a multivitamin as insurance. Not all vitamin supplements are equal. Look for one that has 10 to 12 vitamins and 10 to 12 minerals that meet the recommended daily allowances (RDA). Generic or store brands are often as good as the so-called premium brands and are lower priced. Research has shown that vitamin C, vitamin E, beta-carotene, and selenium are all antioxidants that reduce the damage to tissue from toxic substances called free radicals. Some suggest that vitamins C and E may slow the progression of PD, but research does not confirm this theory. The role of antioxidants in treating PD is unclear.

Get plenty of calcium. PD often strikes people over fifty, those most at risk for bone-thinning osteoporosis and related bone fractures. In addition, if you restrict your protein by cutting down on dairy products to increase the absorption of certain antiparkinson drugs, you may not be getting all the calcium you need. Be sure to get 1,000 to 1,500 milligrams of calcium each day.

Get plenty of fiber. Fiber, the indigestible parts of plants, may help prevent constipation. You may get fiber in your diet from whole grains, fruits, and vegetables.

Drink plenty of water. Water is one of the most important elements of good nutrition. It aids in many processes in the body, including digestion, absorption of nutrients, blood circulation, and excretion of toxins and waste. Drinking plenty of water also enhances the absorption of medication and decreases the risk of dehydration. Unfortunately, our sense of thirst diminishes with age. Also, antiparkinson drugs may dry out the body. Rather than waiting until you're thirsty, drink by the clock. Make sure you drink at least 6 to 8 8-ounce glasses of water per day. Don't count beverages such as coffee, tea, cola, or other caffeinated drinks, which only make you pass more water.

Control nausea. Nausea from both the disease and from antiparkinson medications is common. Walking helps nausea, probably because it helps food move more easily through the di-

> *Listening is essential. When the patient is slow to speak words, don't put words in his mouth. Have patience. Give him the opportunity to communicate his feelings.*
> *Nancy, 36*
> *Speech therapist*

gestive tract. Eating smaller meals, drinking a bit of ginger ale, or drinking ginger tea may help. (To make ginger tea, steep several peeled pieces of fresh ginger in hot water for an hour, then strain and serve.) Drinking a glass of juice or eating a bowl of cereal with a nonprotein, nondairy creamer is also helpful.

Sit down, eat slowly, and chew thoroughly. Avoid eating on the run. It's bad for digestion and may cause you to inhale food into your airways. Eating more slowly and chewing each mouthful thoroughly will aid digestion.

Overcoming Sleep Problems

Getting a good night's sleep can be a problem for anyone. Even among healthy adults, sleep difficulties increase gradually after age thirty-five and are especially bothersome for elderly people. Sleep problems are also common among people with PD. Not only do chronic sleep problems leave one feeling fatigued, they may also aggravate PD symptoms. Common PD-related sleep difficulties include

- waking several times during the night
- waking early in the morning and being unable to get back to sleep
- nightmares
- daytime sleepiness

Some PD-related sleep problems are caused by changes in the brain, nervous system, and muscular changes brought on by the disease. For instance, researchers have found that levels of the brain chemical serotonin, important for deep sleep, are lower in people with PD. Other scientists speculate that sleep problems may be related to changes in the autonomic nervous system. Difficulty falling asleep may be related to depression, persistent tremors, nighttime leg cramping, and restless legs syndrome—

sensations of tingling or pulling in the legs. Nighttime awakenings may also be caused by the reemergence of tremors as medications wear off. Or rigidity and the inability to turn over may cause a person to wake during the night. Early-morning awakenings may occur as medications wear off or from depression and anxiety. Nightmares, vivid dreaming, thrashing, and sleep walking/talking may appear as side effects of levodopa. Some people with PD have difficulties sleeping at night because their sleep-wake cycles have reversed as the result of napping during the day.

I don't have problems falling asleep, but I wake frequently during the night. I have vivid dreams and nightmares and often end up shouting, kicking, or punching wildly in bed. I often wake in the morning not feeling rested, and I feel sleepy during the day.

People tend to internalize their feelings because they don't think anyone understands. Support groups help a lot because they expose you to people who are going through the same things.

Charlene, 47
Clinic Manager

Sleep disturbances may pose problems not only for you but also for your partner and/or caregiver. Interrupted sleep may leave you both exhausted, lacking the reserve energy you need for effectively coping with PD. If your sleep problems are mild to moderate, the following tips may help you get a better night's sleep. If you don't find these suggestions helpful, talk to your physician about medications that may help with sleep.

Accept that you need less sleep. As we age, we need less sleep. If you love to sleep, you may have more difficulty adjusting to this new truth.

Break up your sleep. Don't be afraid to break your sleep into two periods—a short nap in the afternoon and a longer stretch at night.

Avoid oversleeping. Sleep only as much as you need to wake feeling refreshed. Too much sleep, which is often a symptom of depression, may leave you feeling unrested.

Go to bed and get up at the same time every day. Sticking to a schedule helps regulate your internal clock that in turn regulates your sleep-wake cycle.

> *Losing my independence was the most difficult thing, especially not being able to drive. You must realize that you have limitations when the safety of yourself or others is at risk. I still get to where I need to be with the help of my family.*
>
> *Charles*
> *Age 73*

Exercise regularly. Regular, moderate exercise deepens sleep. Sporadic exercising doesn't improve sleep quality. Don't exercise right before going to bed. Make sure you finish your exercise routine at least an hour before going to bed.

Turn down the sound. Many people are light sleepers, easily disturbed by noises. Wear ear-plugs or turn on a fan or white-noise sound machine to muffle external sounds.

Darken the room. Even small amounts of light may disturb sleep. Try using heavy curtains or shades to block out light.

Sleep cool. Rooms that are too warm may disturb sleep. Turn down the furnace and crack a window for fresh air to keep your bedroom at a comfortable sleeping temperature.

Avoid caffeine. Many people have difficulty sleeping after they ingest coffee, tea, cola, or other beverages or foods containing caffeine. If you need a warm drink before bed, try a warm herbal tea or warm milk. Milk contains tryptophan, which helps induce sleep.

Limit alcohol. For some people, a glass of wine or other alcoholic beverage helps them fall asleep. But alcohol also tends to fragment sleep and may cause "rebound" awakenings. If you consume alcohol, do so several hours before retiring.

Avoid liquids after 6:00 P.M. Many people are awakened during the night by a full bladder. If this commonly happens to you, avoid the warm milk remedy and other drinks in the evening. Also, be sure to urinate right before going to bed.

Eat a snack. Hunger may interfere with sleep. Try crackers and cheese, a piece of toast, or warm milk and honey to take the edge off hunger and help induce sleep. Carbohydrates may help calm you and make you sleepy.

Stop smoking. Cigarette, pipe, and cigar smoking are bad for your general health. Chronic tobacco use may also disturb sleep.

Watch what you watch. Television programs or videos with violence or cliff-hanging excitement won't likely put you in the mood to sleep.

Reserve your bed for sleep. Some sleep experts recommend only sleeping in bed. Reading, watching television, doing crossword puzzles, finishing paperwork, and other activities should be reserved for the living room or den. That way, when you get into bed, your mind associates your bed only with sleep.

> *I used to have a hard time holding onto the soap in the shower. Since my husband bought me a nifty soap sock to hang inside the shower, I don't have to bend over and risk falling anymore.*
>
> *Marcia*
> *Age 64*

Try separate beds. If you're rested in the morning but your partner isn't, try separate beds or bedrooms. Often PD-related nightmares, shouting, or thrashing will disturb your partner's sleep more than your own.

Ask about adjusting your medications. If PD symptoms wake you up or if you have to be awake in order to turn over, talk with your doctor. Find out if your medications may be adjusted to better control your symptoms at night.

Go with the flow. If you can't sleep, don't fight it. Get up and read, watch TV, or do some other activity until you feel sleepy.

Try a sleep aid. After two nights of poor sleep, you might consider taking a prescribed sleep medication. Talk with your doctor first.

> *If I wake during the night, I stay in bed in hopes of falling back to sleep. However, if I don't go back to sleep within a reasonable period of time, I get up and read, use my new computer, write, or watch television. Some of my best ideas come in the middle of the night. Usually, I can fall asleep again within an hour.*

Coping with Speech/Swallowing Difficulties

Experts estimate that 60 to 90 percent of people with PD have speech difficulties. Sometimes these problems are quite subtle. Other times, they are debilitating. About half of those with PD have some problem with swallowing.

Speech and swallowing are complex processes that involve many nerves and muscles of the lower face, lips, tongue, voice box, and throat. Just as the automatic muscle movements involved in walking may be affected by PD, so may the automatic muscle and nerve functions involved in speaking and swallowing. In addition, speech and swallowing may be interrupted by unwanted, involuntary movements of the tongue and jaw.

PD-related speech problems occur when the disease affects cells in the brain that regulate muscles in the face and mouth. Doctors call this *hypokinetic dysarthria.* To the listener, it sounds like weak, slow, or uncoordinated talking. It's important to recognize that while this brain problem affects speech, it does not affect intelligence, memory, or personality. It simply affects a person's ability to express him/herself verbally.

While PD-related speech problems are unique to each individual, there are several common complaints. Some people have just one of these problems, while others have multiple speech difficulties.

Hoarseness or breathy voice. As the vocal cords are affected and become stiff and slow, the voice may become hoarse, gravelly, or breathy. This may be an early sign of further speech difficulties.

Loss of volume. This, too, may be one of the first symptoms of PD-related speech problems. It is caused by rigidity and/or stiffness in the breathing muscles. Exhaled breath is the power behind our voices. When muscles in the chest walls are rigid, they cause the exhaled breath to become shallow or irregular. In addition, the breathing muscles lose their elasticity, which normally allows for ever-changing force and speed of breath.

After my diagnosis, I went into a shell. One day I could hardly get out of bed and I panicked because I wanted to live again. I made a remarkable comeback after six months of hard work and determination. People who see me now can't believe it's me.

Stewart
Age 66

Difficulty changing volume. Modifying volume allows us to speak softly or loudly. With PD, some people lose the ability to change volume.

Pitch problems. We change the pitch or melody of our voices to express our thoughts and feelings in ways that go beyond our words. The old adage "how you say something counts" applies here. PD-related speech problems may affect a person's ability to change pitch, resulting in a monotonic voice.

Fast/slow speech. Talking too rapidly or too slowly may be a problem.

Poor pronunciation. Some people with speech difficulties have poor pronunciation. Their words may sound sloppy, run together, or be omitted altogether. It may sound as if the speaker mumbles. This may be caused by changes in the ability of the tongue and lips to move.

If you have any of the speech impairments listed above, it's important that you see a speech therapist immediately. The sooner your speech problems are diagnosed and treated, the better the results.

Each person's speech problems are unique. You will need to be evaluated by a professional speech therapist, preferably a speech-language pathologist who is certified and licensed in treating speech problems. Ask your doctor for a referral to a qualified speech therapist. Or ask a nurse, your physical therapist, other healthcare team member, or local hospital. If you can't find a local referral, write or call the American Speech, Language and Hearing Association (ASLHA) in Rockville, Maryland, for a referral to a speech expert in your area.

A speech therapist will assist you in improving the function of affected muscles, provide exercises that will slow the onset of future speech problems, and, if needed, provide you with other coping strategies and techniques to compensate for losses in your ability to communicate. Not everyone achieves the same results with speech therapy. The effectiveness of speech therapy depends on how quickly help is sought, the motivation of the person, family support, age, and overall health. People with mild, subtle speech changes may expect therapy to return them to normal or almost normal speech. Those with moderate speech problems usually make some gains in speech and learn ways to compensate for problems in being understood. Those with severe problems who are unable to make their needs known with speech can get help with alternative ways of communicating, often with a machine or voice-output computer.

If you have speech problems, in addition to the strategies offered by your therapist, try these tips:

- Be aware of your voice problem and work on it every day. Use a tape recorder to make yourself aware of subtle speech changes.
- Take a deep breath before speaking so that your words come out more forcefully and more clearly.
- Open your mouth to let the sound out.
- Use shorter sentences.
- Clearly enunciate syllables as professional radio announcers do. Exaggerate every sound in every syllable.
- Exercise your voice by reading aloud, shouting, or singing.
- In front of a mirror, practice expressing emotions with your face muscles. Show anger, happiness, sorrow, surprise.
- Let your listeners know about your speech difficulty. If your voice is soft or difficult to understand, ask them to let you know when they can't hear or understand you.

Your speech therapist will likely give you a number of exercises, depending on your particular speech difficulties. The following exercises, recommended by national PD organizations such as the National Parkinson Foundation and the Parkinson's Disease Foundation, may help you reduce muscle rigidity and regain control of the muscles involved in speech. Do the exercises below in front of a mirror daily. (Many of these exercises also help correct swallowing difficulties.)

Deep breathing. Take five deep breaths, stretching out the stomach muscles as you inhale, tightening them as you exhale. Exhale fully, as long as you can, before taking the next breath.

Because patients have troubles swallowing, the Heimlich procedure is something every caregiver should learn. You may doubt your ability to do it, but when you have to, God will give you the strength and courage to save a life.
Marcia
Age 47

Vowel breathing. Take five deep breaths, adding vowel sounds such as "ah," "oh," and "oo" as you exhale.

Automatic speech. Practice reciting strings of words such as the days of the week, months of the year, the alphabet. Be sure to provide good breath support for your words. Pause as needed. Take additional breaths as needed.

Mouth stretch. Open and close your mouth five times, stretching your mouth as much as possible.

Wide smile. Smile five times, stretching your lips back as far as possible.

Nonsense syllables. Smile widely and say "ma, ma, me, me" and "ma, me, mi, mo."

Even syllables. Now try saying "puh puh, puh" ten times. Repeat each syllable evenly and slowly. If you have a metronome to keep time, use it. Say the syllables quickly and evenly. Repeat the instructions above using "tah tah tah," then "kuh kuh kuh," and finally "puh tuh kuh," ten times each.

Tongue out. Stick your tongue out five times. Make it come straight out of your mouth.

Tongue push-ups. Stick out your tongue and push it against the back of a spoon. Repeat five times.

Tongue movement. Move your tongue from side to side and back and forth five times.

Kiss. Pucker your lips as if to kiss a child five times. (Then kiss your caregiver five times!)

Swallowing difficulties, or *dysphagia,* may be more serious than speech problems. Dysphagia may cause life-threatening *aspiration,* the passage of food or drink into the airways. Swallowing seems like a simple enough task, but it's actually quite complicated, involving many nerves and muscles acting simultaneously. PD may affect regions of the brain that detect the presence of food in the mouth or throat, or it may affect the muscles involved in swallowing. Some people with swallowing problems can't feel when food or liquid goes down the wrong way or gets stuck in the throat. This may lead to liquid entering the air pipe, which may in turn cause an infection or lead to pneumonia. Or if a piece of food becomes lodged in the airway, it may cause a life-threatening choking episode.

In addition, swallowing problems may lead to nutrition problems if eating becomes too difficult or unpleasant. Also, not being able to easily eat and enjoy food may cause some people with PD-related swallowing problems to withdraw from social situations.

Signs of Swallowing Problems

Some people with PD have swallowing difficulties and aren't even aware of it. If you or someone you love has PD, be on the lookout for the signs listed below and get help quickly.

- coughing or throat clearing while eating or after a meal
- waking at night, coughing
- changes in voice quality, especially a wet or gurgling sound
- long periods needed to eat a meal
- difficulty eating
- weight loss or dehydration
- beverages are required to wash down foods
- complaints that foods or liquids get stuck in the throat or go down the wrong way
- fever
- pneumonia

When you go in for diagnosis, a speech pathologist will evaluate your swallowing as you eat various foods and beverages. He/she may also do an X-ray study involving barium that allows the pathologist to see the muscles and other structures involved in swallowing. Depending on your problem, the pathologist will then develop an individualized program for you. Your program may include instructions to eat when you are in an "on" period, when your medications are providing maximum benefit, making it easier to swallow.

Dealing with Vision Changes

It is not uncommon for people with PD to complain about vision changes. Some say their vision is blurred. Others have problems focusing and reading. Still others vaguely complain that their eyes are bothering them. Often people with PD visit their eye doctors for changes in glasses or contacts, only to be told their corrected vision is perfect.

Another common vision problem is dry eyes. This may be a side effect of some antiparkinson medications. More often, it is caused by disease-related, infrequent blinking. Frequent use of artificial tears can usually resolve this problem.

Some people with PD complain of eye-muscle fatigue. Often the fatigue is worse on one side. It may cause double vision. Anticholinergics may aggravate these and other eye problems. If you experience eye problems, talk with your doctor. You may need to change your medication.

Can you drive if you have PD? It's an important question many newly diagnosed people ask. For many, driving an automobile represents freedom and independence. Not being able to drive may signal increased dependence that can lead to isolation and depression for those not ready to cope with this change in their lives.

Early in your disease when your symptoms are mild, you will likely still be able to drive. However, as symptoms progress, driving safely may no longer be possible. Muscle rigidity and impaired coordination may impair your ability to make split-second decisions and react quickly, possibly endangering you, your passengers, and others on the road. If you have questions about your ability to continue driving, talk with your doctor.

I prescribe a support group to all of my patients. There are so many things both patients and caregivers can learn from the experiences of others. The camaraderie and socialization alone is a great therapy.

Alex, 53
MD

For those whose disease is well controlled, driving may continue to be a pleasure. If you feel you can still drive safely, follow these commonsense tips:

- Whenever possible ask someone else to drive, or use public transportation.
- Don't drive if you feel fatigued or unstable.
- Don't drive if you have consumed any alcohol. A small amount of alcohol may impair even healthy drivers. Drinking alcohol may also interfere with or dangerously interact with your medications. Talk with your doctor about alcoholic beverages and your medications.
- Avoid driving after sunset. Even healthy adults have difficulty seeing well in the dark.

Dealing with Sexuality Issues

Sexual desire and sexual performance are highly individual. Later in life, some men and women have less sexual desire. For some older men, sexual dysfunction—especially difficulty achieving and maintaining an erection—is a problem. After menopause, some women experience a marked decrease in sexual desire. For most, PD comes later in life and coincides with a decline in sexual interest and/or activity. Many men and women, however, remain sexually interested and active well into their later years.

For most of us, our sexual relationships are central to who we are. We are sexual beings. Sexual relationships fill basic biological needs. Moreover, a satisfying sexual relationship may fulfill our need for intimacy, closeness, touch, pleasure. It may help us release tension and connect with another human being.

Little information is available about the impact of PD on sexuality. Experts do know that PD affects the autonomic nervous system. As a result, it impacts one's response to sexual stimulation. In addition, PD inhibits agility and the ability to move freely. It may impair one's ability to express emotions, cause incontinence and bowel problems, and shrink unused muscles. Many antiparkinson drugs decrease sexual desire and diminish sexual functioning. Less commonly, antiparkinson dopamine medications result in hypersexuality, mild to severe increases in sexual desire and interest accompanied by vivid dreams and sleep disturbances.

For men, the changes they experience in sexual function may be related as much to aging as they are to PD. The male sex hormone testosterone begins diminishing after age 25. By age 50, achieving an erection takes two to three times longer than at age 35 or 40. Often a full erection cannot be achieved until just before climax. Not only does it take longer to get an erection, the erection may disappear quickly after orgasm. As arteries narrow with aging, the flow of blood to the penis is decreased or blocked, making erection difficult and/or impossible.

> *Hope and faith help me to endure the things that I really don't understand.*
>
> *Chris*
> *Age 77*

In men with PD, changes in the autonomic nervous system may interfere with the brain's signal to the penis for erection. Drugs taken for PD or other health problems may hamper erection. Bladder and bowel problems, especially incontinence, may also impact sexual function.

Erection difficulties and other sexual problems may have a huge impact on a man's sense of self. Men have been raised to believe that sexual prowess is an indicator of manhood. The inability to achieve and maintain an erection and "perform" sexually is seen by most men as the ultimate humiliation. For men with PD who have already been robbed of many traditional male roles, sexuality problems may have a tremendous negative impact on their self-esteem.

Most women with PD have undergone or are undergoing menopause. This major life change causes the clitoris to shrink, decreases normal lubrication in the vagina, and makes the vaginal walls thinner and less elastic, which can make intercourse painful and/or less satisfying. In addition, some women experience changes in sexual desire with menopause. Some have more desire, while others have less or almost none.

There are times I need my cane; however, I try to do everything I can without it. When I have it with me I feel more confident and secure and that is important.
Randall
Age 64

Fluctuations in the female hormones progesterone and estrogen may make some antiparkinson medications work less effectively or quit working altogether. For most women, the problems occur just before menses every month. Postmenopausal women, too, may experience hormone fluctuations that produce similar problems with antiparkinson medications.

Some women have difficulty experiencing orgasms. PD impedes autonomic nerve responses and muscle movement, both important in sexual response. Drugs for PD and other health problems may make achieving orgasm problematic. As with men, bowel and bladder problems may also negatively impact sexual desire and functioning.

On an emotional level, PD may attack a woman's belief in her femininity. As the disease progresses, a woman may see herself as less attractive, less desirable, and less able to be a fulfilling sexual partner.

There are plenty of things you and your partner can do to improve your sex life.

Get your disease under control. A balanced drug regimen is the best treatment for PD symptoms that can impact sexuality. In addition, it is important to employ all the self-help strategies you can to lessen the impact of your symptoms on your sexuality, including exercising regularly, getting enough rest, managing stress, and eating a well-balanced diet.

Try satin sheets. They make turning over in bed easier and can improve agility.

Plan sex for "on" times. Some people object to planning sexual activity, claiming it takes the spontaneity out of sex. However, spontaneity is not necessary for sexual satisfaction. Planning seduction—and timing it so that it coincides with times when your antiparkinson drugs are most effective—may actually increase anticipation and sexual pleasure.

Renew romance. Couples who have been together for a long time may have lost the romance and passion of their early years. PD may complicate this further, especially as the disease progresses. For someone with PD, the symptoms and physical limitations may make it difficult to feel sexual. For an exhausted caregiver, sexual activity may be the last thing on his or her mind. For some lucky couples, the challenges of PD bring them even closer together. Others are not so lucky. If sexuality issues are a problem for you and your mate, you may want to seek the help of a skilled therapist.

Going to support group meetings allowed me to interact with other caregivers who understand. They gave me suggestions and ideas that really helped me through the rough spots.

Patty
Age 52

Talk about it. Honest communication and trying to understand and respond to one another's needs are the keys to a mutually satisfying relationship, no matter your age or physical condition. Ask for what you need sexually.

Get help. All of us carry some psychological issues concerning sex. Combine these with a chronic illness, and the result may prove disastrous. If your efforts to improve your communication and your sex life aren't enough, try talking with a mental health therapist. A skilled therapist can often help couples work through even the most difficult issues.

If Incontinence Is a Problem

- *Get evaluated by a urologist.* It's the only way to find out what is causing the problem.
- *Ask about changing medications.* Sometimes bowel and bladder problems are side effects of medications.
- *Women can practice Kegel exercises.* Ask your doctor about these exercises which may improve muscle tone in the vagina, control the urinary outlet, and help prevent urine leakage. During these exercises, a woman squeezes and releases the muscles in the vaginal area as if to stop the flow of urine. These contractions can be performed throughout the day—while driving, sitting, lying down.
- *Drink plenty of water.* Drink eight to ten glasses of water or juice daily to help you stay healthy and regular.
- *Limit beverages at night.*
- *Try grapefruit juice and coffee.* Both stimulate urination to help you empty your bladder.
- *Talk to your doctor about water pills.* Taking a diuretic medication in the morning may help prevent incontinence.

- *Don't wait until you feel the urge to urinate.* Women in particular have been taught to "hold it" rather than urinating when the urge strikes. Take every opportunity to empty your bladder.
- *Urinate before sexual activity.* It will help prevent urine spillage during climax.
- *Eat roughage.* If constipation is a problem, eat lots of fiber. Fruits, vegetables, and bran are high in fiber.
- *Exercise regularly.* It helps relieve constipation and improves overall physical and mental health.

Decreasing Dizziness/Fainting

Some people with PD suffer from low blood pressure, or *orthostatic hypotension*. Those with very low blood pressure may experience dizziness, fainting, fatigue, unsteadiness, or slowing of mental processes. It is often most noticeable when you rise from a sitting or lying position. You may feel lightheaded or dizzy. The following tips may be helpful:

Do a medication check. Talk with your doctor about stopping any unnecessary medications. Sometimes low blood pressure is a side effect of certain drugs. Nearly all antiparkinson drugs may produce this side effect. Also talk to your physician about medications that may help with the low blood pressure.

Drink water. Drink at least eight glasses a day to replenish body fluids.

Try wearing thigh-high elastic stockings. They can help prevent pooling of blood in the lower legs.

Take care when rising from a sitting or lying position. Take your time and get up slowly. Fatigue and sitting for long periods in a warm bath or other warm environment are definitely aggravating factors. Have someone at your side when you stand up. Sit or lie down immediately if you feel the symptoms coming on.

Calming Restless Legs

Restless legs syndrome (RLS) is a motor movement disorder, creating uncomfortable sensations in the legs. Some people describe RLS as feeling like a pulling, tingling, or aching in the legs. Others describe a need to move their legs. The exact cause of the disorder is not known.

RLS comes on when one is inactive, with symptoms usually becoming worse during sleep. Bouts of movements in one or both legs may disturb one's sleep. Even if the sleeper isn't fully awakened by these movements, he/she may wake feeling tired.

Although rubbing or moving the legs immediately may relieve the discomfort, the sensation usually returns within seconds. Doctors don't know what causes most cases of RLS. If you have RLS, ask your attending physician how medications may help. Some individuals may get relief from a combination of carbidopa and levodopa; others report good results with one of the dopamine agonists. Sometimes a hot, soothing bath helps.

Staying Safe and Comfortable at Home

More than 90 percent of people with PD live at home with loved ones. Home is where most of us feel comfortable and safe. However, home may also become a dangerous place if the right adaptations aren't made to accommodate the changes caused by PD. (See Resources for companies that offer adaptive aids.)

Preventing Falls. Falls are the most common accidental injury in the home. Anyone who is ill, injured, frail, or elderly is especially at risk. Falls present a major hazard for those with PD. In addition, many older people with PD have lost calcium in their bones, making them even more vulnerable to serious injury. Making a few simple changes around the house may help prevent falls.

Make walkways safe. Tack down and/or remove loose carpets and throw rugs. Remove raised doorsills. Move furniture out of walkways. Make sure all furniture with sharp edges or corners is removed. Install handrails adjacent to entryways and in hallways. Take valuable, breakable objects out of harm's way.

Make stairs safe. Make sure stairways have sturdy railings. Repair cracked steps, loose handrails, or other problem areas that may cause falls. Install colored strips of tape on steps to make them more visible.

Increase lighting. Install soft, nonglare, incandescent 100-watt bulbs above staircases and 75-watt bulbs in hallways. Shade bulbs to prevent excess glare. Place night-lights where appropriate. Install motion lights—they automatically light up your way as you pass by.

Make bathrooms safe. Install grab bars next to the toilet and in the shower and bathtub. Use rubber mats in the shower and bathtub. Make sure the toilet is the right height. A raised toilet seat, available at home-care supply stores, makes rising from the toilet easier and safer.

Making Meals Enjoyable

With slowness and chewing and swallowing problems, many people with PD find mealtimes frustrating. Also, lack of coordination may make cooking meals difficult, even dangerous. A few adaptations will help you enjoy meals.

Take the time you need. It will take longer for you to cook and eat. Take your time. Chew your food thoroughly. If your food gets cold, use an electric warming tray. Others at your table can use the time to sit around the table and enjoy one another's company.

Have your meat cut. Handling a knife may be a problem. Having your meat precut should make it easier.

Choose utensils that work. Use a spoon instead of a fork, if it's easier. Home health-aid stores offer special utensils with thicker handles that make grasping easier.

Try straws. Tremors may make drinking difficult. A flexible straw should help.

> *There is a lot both physical and occupational therapists can do to keep patients safe, mobile and independent. Seek help in making accommodations in your home and take advantage of tools that can make daily activities easier.*
>
> *Carol, 33*
> *Physical therapist*

Choose large-handled mugs, especially if grasping is difficult.

Alter the texture. Try preparing your food in a food processor or blender. Thick soups or stews are often easier to eat.

Eat smaller meals more often. It is easier to digest smaller amounts of food. Smaller, more frequent meals will also help you maintain a constant supply of energy throughout the day. Try eating a light breakfast, a mid-morning snack, a light lunch, a midafternoon snack, a moderate dinner, and a light meal in the evening.

Use helpful kitchen aids. Cooking may be easier if you use kitchen aids such as jar openers, cutting boards with suction cups and lips to prevent food from slipping off, reachers to grasp items in cupboards or pick up dropped items, and pot stabilizers to keep pots and pans from sliding off the stove. Electric can openers are also convenient. Sometimes a microwave oven is safer and more convenient than a stove.

Dressing/Grooming Made Easier

PD may impair the fine motor coordination and strength required for dressing and grooming. A few adaptations may help you maintain your independence in these very personal tasks.

Wear shoes with Velcro strips instead of laces. Or buy elastic shoelaces that can be permanently tied so that you can simply slip shoes on and off.

Replace buttons with zippers or other fasteners that are easier to use. Large zipper pulls or rings make opening and closing garments easier. For blouse or shirt cuffs, sew on buttons with elastic thread that allows you to slip your hand through without unbuttoning.

Choose loose, stretchy clothing. It's easier to get on and off.

Enlarge armholes. Coat sleeves may be too narrow to get your arm into easily. Have a tailor widen the armholes by two inches so that you may put on your coat without assistance.

Try a front-closing bra. They are often easier to close than back-closing bras.

Use a long-handled shoehorn and a sock donner. They may prevent straining when you put on socks and shoes.

Turn up the heat. The fewer clothes the better for many people with PD. Turn the heat up a bit to avoid putting on more clothes.

Use an electric shaver to avoid cuts from razors. Holders for electric razors are also available, if needed.

Try a suction nailbrush to make grooming easier. It may be secured to the tub.

Use soap on a rope. This keeps soap conveniently within reach.

Try a long-handled brush or sponge for bathing.

Replace tub faucet handles. Try single-arm control levers to make them easier to operate.

Other Helpful Aids

Books on tape. They provide excellent entertainment, especially for tired eyes.

Bed pulls. Bed pulls may be attached to the side or the end of a bed frame or to assist with turning. They may be purchased or made by braiding three pieces of fabric together. Bed pulls should be long enough to reach from the side or end of the bed to your hands when you're lying down. Attach large, wooden curtain rings on the ends as handles.

Trapeze. A triangular-shaped handle may be installed over the head of your bed to make it easier to change positions.

Urinals. Kept within easy reach, they can eliminate nighttime walks to the bathroom.

> *The tenacity and internal strength I see in some patients is amazing. Sometimes I wonder if that were me, whether I would be that positive or enthusiastic.*
>
> *Cynthia, 35*
> *Physical therapist*

Wedge cushions. These may make sitting up in bed easier.

Bed rails. These may help you turn over and get out of bed. Bed rails may be installed on the wall near your bed or attached to your bed frame.

Tub seats or shower chairs. These may make bathing or showering easier.

A hand-held shower hose. These devices will allow you to sit while bathing.

Making Travel Easier

PD may make travel more difficult, but not impossible. If you love to travel, don't give it up. With a little help, travel can still be part of your life.

- Traveling with a companion will make your trip easier and, in many cases, more fun.
- Ask for help. While it is important to be as independent as possible, it is equally important to ask for help when you need it and let people know exactly what assistance you need. Employees in the travel industry are accustomed to providing help for customers who need it. Don't be afraid to ask. Bellhops can handle your luggage. Waiters are happy to cut your meat in the kitchen. Airline personnel will gladly preboard you onto a plane.
- Take extra medication and copies of your prescriptions. Be sure to carry these aboard rather than checking them with your baggage.
- Wear a Medic-Alert bracelet. It will alert medical personnel in the event of a medical emergency.

8

Caring for Caregivers

When your partner or other significant person in your life develops PD, he/she isn't the only one affected. Everyone in the family is impacted by the disease, especially caregivers. Caregiving is a difficult task—emotionally, spiritually, and physically. While caregiving is an expression of love for someone who is important to you, it is also frustrating, lonely, isolating, and at times overwhelming even for the strongest and most dedicated people. This chapter is for caregivers, the foot soldiers in the fight against PD.

At its best, caregiving is a mutual relationship. True, one partner may give more than the other. A health crisis such as PD may actually strengthen the bonds and intimacy a couple shares. At its worst, caregiving may breed resentment and anger. Both may feel overwhelmed but fearful of asking for outside help. As more demands are placed on the caregiver and the roles of each person changes, the relationship may be strained to the breaking point.

Coping with Emotional Challenges

Learning your partner or loved one has PD means changing the lifestyle you shared together and embarking on a life you didn't bargain for. It means a future that is uncertain in many respects and all too certain in others. Confusing and conflicting feelings are likely to come up—anger, sadness, hopelessness, resentment. It is difficult to deal with so-called "negative" feelings. We're not "supposed" to have those feelings. But we do. Somehow we feel guilty for having them.

Perhaps you'll identify with some of the common feelings, listed below, mentioned by those who have experienced the frustration that can come with caregiving.

Anger. "Sometimes I feel trapped. I struggle with feelings of anger and guilt."

Sadness. "I've lost a healthy spouse to a chronic, disabling, incurable disease. We had so much to look forward to."

Loneliness. "Everybody wants to know how he's feeling. No one even asks about me."

Guilt. "I sometimes feel ashamed of my feelings. Why do I have to take on this unwelcome problem?"

Resentment. "I didn't ask for this burden. Why me?"

Hopelessness. "Everything has changed, and you realize your lives will never be the same again."

Loss of intimacy. "We don't communicate well. We're less intimate. How do I say that I'm scared and feel deprived?"

Unfortunately, in caregiving someone with PD, your needs and feelings may take second place to those of your ill loved one. There are plenty of things you can do to help yourself cope with the emotional aspects of caregiving.

Give yourself permission to feel your feelings. Feelings are neither good nor bad. They're just feelings. Accept that many so-called negative feelings such as sadness, anger, frustration, guilt, and resentment are all part of caregiving. Allow yourself to recognize all your feelings and let go of your guilt.

Learn effective ways to release difficult emotions. Exercise, talking with supportive friends and family members, meditation, writing in your journal, and stress reduction techniques are all good ways to let go of negative feelings.

> *Whenever I have a difficult day, I keep reminding myself that for seventy of my 77 years I did not have PD. Not a bad average. Meanwhile, thanks to a very unselfish caregiver, I lead a pretty good life. In fact I don't have enough time to do the things I can and want to do.*
>
> *Link*
> *Age 77*

Channel your feelings into constructive behavior. You're feeling angry and frustrated. You call the doctor, yell, and hang up. Or you scream at your children, kick the dog, or throw and break a lovely, prized plate. None of these is an effective coping strategy. Your feelings aren't the problem. It's how you act out those feelings that counts. Try rechanneling your anger and frustration into forming a support group for caregivers, finding the community services you need, or raising money for PD research.

Recognize and get help for depression. The losses associated with PD and the demands placed on you may cause you to sink into depression. You may need professional help.

Talk about your feelings. You need to talk with your doctor, your loved one, your friends, family, and/or members of your PD support group about your feelings.

Put your anger where it belongs. Anger, resentment, and blaming can spill over to your ill loved one and/or to other friends and family members. Instead, get angry with the disease. Give yourself permission to blame the illness for your troubles. It frees you from blaming yourself and/or your partner for things that are beyond your control.

Accept that to give is also to receive. There are many gifts you get back as a caregiver, including feelings of pride, joy, relief, love, and commitment.

Find something to do while you allow your partner the time to accomplish those things he/she can still do. Listen to music, read, knit, or answer mail so you don't feel as though you are wasting time.

Learn relaxation techniques. Meditation, progressive relaxation, visualization, and bio-feedback may help.

Practice positive self-talk. Instead of telling yourself how bad things are, tell yourself that you can do this, that you have success-fully faced many challenges before.

Become involved in a support group. If your community doesn't have a caregiver sup-port group, start one. Talk with your doctor, your hospital, or mental health agency for help. Or, if you are on-line, look for a care-giver chat group.

Don't be afraid to laugh. Every difficult situation has its hu-mor. Taking a lighter approach may reduce stress and help you face difficult times.

Being diagnosed with Parkinson's disease has given me a greater appreciation for life. I pay more attention to details now, which has enabled me to see a whole new world of beauty. I am thankful for having the chance to look at life in this way.

John
Age 70

Take time for yourself. You deserve to have pleasure and joy in your life. You must nourish yourself, take time for yourself, care for yourself. If you want to be there for your loved one, you must give yourself time-outs to pursue other interests and relationships. Ask family and friends if they can take over caregiving duties occasionally so that you may have a break. See a movie, visit a friend, take up a hobby.

Mobilize friends and family to help. Often we think we should do everything ourselves. However, caring for someone with a chronic illness can be overwhelming, especially over time. Let others know how they can help and gratefully accept their assistance.

> *From my experience with patients, the best thing you can do for someone is just be there.*
>
> *Anne, 48*
> *RN*

Bring in some paid help. If you don't have family support, consider hiring an in-home caregiver or taking your loved one to a day-time care program.

Adjust your expectations. Life won't be normal no matter how much you want it to be. Don't insist on normalcy. Some chores such as dusting, vacuuming, cleaning, and yard work may have to be cut back, eliminated, or delegated to someone else. Life doesn't have to be perfect.

Handling the Spiritual Crisis

For many caregivers, spirituality provides the strength needed to face the challenges of PD. But the rigors of caregiving may bring on a spiritual crisis for both the caregiver and the person with PD. Your spirituality may have led you to believe that everything happens for a reason, according to a plan. Or perhaps you believe that people get what they deserve. Suddenly, your spiritual beliefs are thrown into question. How could God let this happen? You're a good person. Instead of the joys of leisure and retirement, you both now face the uncertainty of a chronic disease. You may ask, "Why me?" You may feel angry that your Higher Power has let you down. You may feel guilty because you think it is a sin to be angry with God. You may even begin to lose your faith.

"Why do bad things happen to good people?" you may ask. Few explanations can make sense of such things. Even if we think we have figured it out, we are still left with pain, anguish, and feelings of unfairness. Perhaps we instead need to ask, "How will I respond?" and "What will I do now?"

If you find your spirituality is waning, find someone to help. Your pastor, rabbi, counselor, or other trusted person can help you gain new perspectives on your situation.

Here are some tips for facing your spiritual challenges:

Accept that you are not in control. It is difficult for most of us to acknowledge that we have little control over many aspects of our lives. Once you accept that, you can regain a sense of balance by looking to the areas where you can feel in control, to those situations that are organized and predictable.

Find pleasure in small wonders. Take time to appreciate a beautiful sunset, a blooming flower, the changing seasons, the laughter of a child.

Keep a grateful journal. Take time each day to write down five things for which you are grateful. They can be as small as the taste of a cup of coffee or as grand as your gratitude for freedom. Record all your grateful observations in your journal.

Reconnect with your spiritual self. Take time each day to meditate, pray, or otherwise connect with that quiet place inside and your higher spiritual power.

Spend time in nature. For many people, walking in the woods is more spiritual than spending time in a church or synagogue. Connecting with nature can awaken you to the miracle that is life.

Change your perspective on caregiving. Instead of seeing caregiving as a burden you must bear, look at it as an opportunity to grow and learn.

See yourself as strong and capable. Take time each day to visualize yourself competently handling all the challenges you face. Try using affirmations such as "I effortlessly handle all the challenges I am presented" or "I have all the resources I need to handle any situation."

Facing the Physical Challenges

PD challenges a caregiver physically. Suddenly, you are faced not only with caring for your ill partner but also with assuming many of your mate's tasks. A husband, for instance, who chopped wood and took care of the yard work before becoming ill may now not be able to do that work. A wife who previously did the cooking, shopping, and housecleaning may have to turn over those tasks to her mate.

Often caregiving means being pushed physically beyond your endurance. You may hurriedly eat meals in front of the refrigerator. You may be fatigued from being awakened at night by a partner who is restless from PD symptoms or medications. Your back may ache from lifting and moving your ill loved one.

It is not uncommon for caregivers to become ill themselves. Research has demonstrated that stress contributes to a host of ailments, including high blood pressure, ulcers, depression and anxiety, and heart disease. To cope with the physical, mental, and emotional challenges of caregiving, you have to take care of yourself physically. Here are some tips:

Manage stress. Try humor, exercise, and relaxation techniques to manage the stress in your life.

Exercise regularly. Keeping physically fit may help reduce the emotional and physical strain. It may also make you stronger and better able to meet the physical demands of caregiving, such as helping a person move from a bed to a wheelchair.

Avoid excessive alcohol. Because it is a depressant, alcohol won't help you cope with your situation. If you find yourself turning to alcohol or other drugs to cope, get some help fast.

Eat a well-balanced diet. A good diet is important for you, too. Eat plenty of whole grains, fruits, and vegetables. Drink six to eight glasses of water per day. Reduce fat, caffeine, alcohol, refined sugar, and salt.

> *For me, the Internet has helped me learn how to cope with this disease. Not only is it a library at my fingertips, but also a way to communicate with people all over the world. It's like a support group in my home.*
>
> *Richard*
> *Age 63*

Get plenty of rest. Lack of rest is a major contributor to depression and exhaustion. People with PD are often erratic sleepers. They may thrash about with vivid dreams, wake frequently, talk in their sleep. This may leave you sleepless and exhausted. As difficult as it may be to accept, it may be time to sleep in separate bedrooms or separate beds.

Learn proper moving, lifting, and transferring techniques. Your loved one may feel humiliated and embarrassed to need assistance moving. However, as the disease progresses, it may be necessary for the caregiver to help the person get into or out of chairs or bed. Using proper body mechanics and the right techniques and equipment may help maintain the ill person's dignity and prevent injuries. Talk with your loved one's doctor and/or physical therapist about good lifting/moving techniques.

- Encourage your loved one to move as independently as possible.
- Allow plenty of time for moving.
- Move the person from their strongest side.
- Think safety to avoid falls. Check personal equipment such as wheelchairs and walkers before using. Lock side rails on beds. Use brakes on wheels of beds, shower chairs, wheelchairs, and commodes.
- Use the right equipment. Safety belts, lifts, and other aids can make lifting easier for you and the person you're moving.
- Use good body mechanics when assisting someone:
  - ✓ Use your legs rather than your back.
  - ✓ Spread your legs to give yourself a wide base of support.
  - ✓ Move your whole body rather than just bending or twisting.
  - ✓ Keep the person close to you.
  - ✓ Avoid jerky movements and lifting whenever possible. Instead, use rolling, pivoting, or sliding to move the person.
  - ✓ Use both arms and get help when you need it.

Getting Help

As PD progresses, so do the demands placed on a caregiver. Many try to shoulder all the emotional and physical burdens alone. Even the best caregiver, for a variety of reasons, may no longer be able to continue caring for his/her loved one without help. Where can you find help?

Friends and family. Let others know exactly what kind of help you need. Perhaps you can work out a schedule so that a relative or friend can stay with your loved one or take him/her for an outing to give you a break.

Your church or synagogue. Sometimes they run senior programs or adult day-care services that can provide help.

Meals on Wheels. If cooking meals becomes difficult on top of all your other responsibilities, social service agencies such as Meals on Wheels can deliver hot meals to your home. Often, these services are available free or at minimal cost.

Community Services. Check your state's Area Office on Aging for a list of the services offered in your community. Also, check in your local phone book under "community services" and "senior services."

Home-care services. These provide either skilled nursing care prescribed by a physician or respite/support services for personal care and household chores. Be sure to shop around before selecting a home-care agency or individual to provide these services. Find out the qualifications of the individual/agency. Be sure to ask:

The best advice I could give caregivers after 13 years experience is: Be sure to save time for your own interests and activities. Letting the patient's needs overwhelm all of yours puts you in danger of depression and burnout which is bad for both of you.

Nancy
Age 70

- their experience working with people with PD.
- whether they are licensed and bonded.
- their references and be sure to check them.
- the fees charged. (Check with your insurance plan to see if any of the services are covered.)

Independence dogs. Special companion dogs are often overlooked by PD caregivers. Independence Dogs, Inc., is a school that specially trains dogs to help people with PD (see Resources). These animals are not only excellent companions for those with PD, they can also provide needed respite for caregivers. The dogs are trained to help the ill person get up after a fall, help with episodes of "freezing," open doors, pick up objects, and perform a variety of other tasks. The cost for a companion dog is a small donation. The person receives three weeks of training with the dog. The demand for the dogs is high, and the waiting list is long. However, with a bit of planning, you can get your loved one signed up for one of these wonderful animals and have it by the time he/she really needs it.

I heard a doctor speak at a seminar about the strides being made in training dogs to help people with movement disorders. So having dogs to help people move safely will be tremendous. If people stay mobile, they'll be independent longer.

Merlin
Age 53

Financial Help

PD could prove financially devastating for any family. As soon as a diagnosis of PD is made, it is important to begin planning. Since each family's financial situation is different, no single formula works for everyone. The key is to plan as far ahead as possible to avoid having to react in a crisis and make poor decisions.

Take a realistic look at your financial situation. Cut down on unnecessary expenditures. If needed, hire a financial consultant, accountant, or lawyer to help. Legal Aid or Consumer Credit Counseling provides help at no cost if you meet income eligibility requirements.

Thoroughly review your health insurance. What is covered? What is not covered? What is the maximum lifetime benefit? Does it cover long-term care? (Note: Medicare does not cover long-term nursing costs.) Will it cover in-home health services? If you don't have health insurance, many states now have insurance pools for those who meet income requirements.

Set up a budget. Be sure to include additional costs for medications, doctor visits, and costs of hospitalization not covered by your insurance.

Explore ways to enhance your family's income and still function as caregiver. Try to stay employed as long as possible.

Contact Social Security. They can tell you about your benefits and eligibility requirements. Numbers are listed in the government section of your phone book.

Contact Medicare. They can help you understand what Medicare does and does not cover. They are listed in the government section of your phone book. Also, under "disability services," look for Centers for Independent Living. These provide assistance for seniors and disabled people, including job counseling and housing assistance.

> *Rather than restricting patients, encourage them to explore their full potentials. As a caregiver, I know how it is to want to provide assistance. But sometimes you can help loved ones more by giving them the freedom to be independent.*
>
> *JoAnn*
> *Age 36*

Get tax help. Provisions in the IRS tax code allow you to deduct medical expenses, including durable medical equipment and modifications to your home or automobile. At present, you may deduct costs for doctors, drugs, equipment, and treatment or therapy if they total more than 7.5 percent of your total income, less some items such as IRA contributions, but before you deduct other items such as home-mortgage interest and charitable contributions. Even modifications to your house are eligible, including ramps, guardrails, and widened doorways. Talk with your accountant or tax advisor about how to make the most of these tax deductions.

Living Will and Durable Power of Attorney

Planned instructions—advance directives—give your loved one the power to decide what treatment he/she wants to receive if and when he/she is no longer able to make those decisions. They also relieve the caregiver and other family members of having to make potentially agonizing decisions. Advance directives need not cost any money to prepare.

Living Will

A living will is a statement made by a person about what he/she wants done in terms of health-care if he/she becomes mentally incapable of making those decisions. A living will is a statement of a person's desire to die with dignity. It usually expresses the individual's wish that no extraordinary life-sustaining measures be taken. An attorney may draw up a living will. You may also use standard forms or make your own. First check your state laws.

Durable Power of Attorney

This document enables an individual to identify someone (often a partner-caregiver) to act as his/her agent if he/she becomes incapacitated. It means the caregiver or other person designated as agent can make needed health-care decisions when the ill person can't make those decisions for him/herself. It also means the ill person can make his or her wishes known at the time the durable power of attorney is drawn up. Be sure to check your state laws regarding this document. Some states require special witnesses and/or restrict who can be appointed agent.

Long-Term Care: Making Difficult Decisions

For some, complications from the disease or other health problems may make it impossible to live at home. Making the decision to place a loved one in a foster home or nursing home can be agonizing for caregivers and their families.

Let's face it, there's no place like home. In the best of all worlds, all of us would end our days in our homes surrounded by loved ones and caregivers with inexhaustible reserves of energy, patience, and time. This isn't always possible. As a caregiver, you may be facing health problems of your own. Other family members may have more energy for caregiving but much less time.

From my observations, one of the biggest issues for patients and caregivers is finding a happy medium between safety and dignity.

Laura, 30
Physical therapist

It may also not be financially feasible to continue caregiving at home. Caregiving at home is less expensive than a care facility, but it is often impossible to find the financial resources to hire the extra help that would make home care possible. Medicaid, for instance, which is available to lower-income families, will pay for full-time nursing home costs but will pay for few home-care costs. Even when it is possible to pay for home care or day care, some people with PD with mental changes are threatened by any change. They may resist new caregivers or refuse to attend day-care programs. They may verbally lash out at their partner-caregiver. Over time, the progression of the disease and impairment of mobility may pose a threat to the person with PD and sometimes the caregiver, too.

Making the decision to place a loved one in a nursing home or other care facility is difficult. You may be torn by your loved one's resistance to leaving home and your need for help. Here are some tips for helping with this transition:

> *I think it's important that, as caretakers, we take good care of ourselves, too. If we burn out, we can be of no help to anyone.*
> *Paul*
> *Age 48*

Plan ahead. Talk with your loved one honestly about the need for care facilities in the future. If possible, visit facilities and make choices before such care is necessary. For some people, it is impossible to face the impending loss of their independence and take these steps. This leaves the caregiver to make these decisions, often alone, and sometimes with criticism from other family members.

Work with your primary care doctor. Your doctor will be key in determining what level of care is needed for your loved one. It is also likely that your doctor has established relationships with one or more care facilities in your area. Ask him/her for recommendations.

Check with your Area Office on Aging. They publish a guide to nursing homes that contains basic information you will need to make an informed choice.

Ask for a Medicare assessment. Call your local Medicare office and ask for a nursing-home admission review. They will determine whether your loved one qualifies for coverage in a skilled-care facility. If you are under your state's insurance plan, staffers for that program can determine eligibility.

Treat the facility as your loved one's home. Once your loved one has been moved to a care facility, make it feel homey. Bring some personal items to make the room feel familiar.

Give it time. Adjustment to a new place may be difficult, especially if your loved one has PD-related mental changes. If the person has memory problems, avoid taking him/her for drives or visits home for at least six weeks or until he/she has accepted the facility as a new home. It may be heart-wrenching to try to convince a confused loved one to go back to the care facility after a visit home.

Develop good relationships. It is important for you and your family to develop a good relationship with the staff of the care facility. Avoid being hypercritical. No matter how good the care facility, it is not home. It is easy to misplace your guilt and become angry with the facility.

Get a feel for the place. Make a habit of visiting the facility at different times of the day. Attend an activity. Eat a meal there. Try not to make snap decisions about the facility, especially during the first few weeks of adjustment.

To determine whether your loved one is receiving good care, ask yourself the following questions:

- How is he/she doing compared with functioning at home?
- Is he/she clean and dry?
- Is he/she being encouraged to be as active as possible?
- Is he/she receiving the individualized care needed to foster mobility, functioning, and personal dignity?
- Is your loved one receiving the right medication in the correct dosage in a timely manner?

If you have concerns, talk with the nurse in charge or the administrator of the facility.

Make sure the staff understands the challenges of PD. Some staff may not have much experience caring for people with PD. Make sure, for instance, that they understand how important it is to administer medications exactly on time and provide opportunities for exercise. If you need help educating the facility staff, talk with your doctor.

9

Hope for the Future

In the last ten years, researcher scientists have made great strides in understanding neurological disorders and how the brain works. They've also learned more about new drugs for treating symptoms of diseases such as PD, creating safer surgical procedures, and developing new treatment strategies, including exciting areas such as gene therapy. There is plenty of reason for optimism about treatment and the eventual cure for PD.

New Drugs

Since the discovery of l-dopa thirty years ago, several new, effective, and powerful antiparkinson drugs have been introduced. Currently, at least thirty new antiparkinson drugs are being tested. Several of the newer drugs not only relieve PD symptoms but may also slow the progression of the disease.

The experimental drug Ro 40-7592, which is being investigated by scientists at the National Institute of Neurological Disorders and Stroke, has shown the ability to increase symptom relief by 60 percent when added to the standard carbidopa/levodopa drug therapy. The drug appears to block the breakdown of dopamine and levodopa, allowing people with PD to take fewer doses and smaller amounts of carbidopa/levodopa.

Research into drugs called *neuroimmunophilins*, which have the ability to rejuvenate nerves and neurons, is also encouraging. Discovered a few years ago by scientists at Johns Hopkins, the drug FK-506 (now marketed as cyclosporine, an immuno-supressant) was the first drug shown to stimulate the growth of brain cells that have been damaged. In animals, the drug helped partially rejuvenate nerves in leg and spinal-cord injuries.

> *What would I say to someone who recently found out they have PD? "You are the lucky ones. With the increased levels of research the probability is high that a satisfactory cure will be available when you really need it."*
>
> *Joe*
> *Age 70*

Brain scientist Solomon Snyder was able to successfully isolate the portion of cyclosporine responsible for the nerve-stimulating effects. He was then able to produce drug-like molecules that mimic these nerve-regenerating effects. When given to animals with PD-like symptoms, these molecules (called GPI-1046) stimulated the regrowth of damaged neurons and eliminated all signs of the disease. GPI-1046 and other neuroimmunophilins may be given orally and are able to cross the blood-brain barrier. Unlike many other medications, these drugs appear to target only damaged nerves, leaving healthy nerves intact. Human trials are to begin soon, but it may be some time before this drug is available.

Other ways of administering drugs are being studied. Scientists are investigating controlled-release formulas of PD drugs and pumps that could be implanted into the body to provide a continuous supply of levodopa. One promising study involves implanting levodopa capsules in the brain. The capsules would release the drug into the brain at a timed rate.

The search for more effective medications to treat PD patients will likely be aided by the recent discovery of at least five different types of brain receptors for dopamine. New information about the unique aspects of each receptor in different areas of the brain has led to new treatment theories and clinical trials for testing new medications.

Gene Therapy

Another promising area of research into the treatment of PD is *gene therapy*. A gene carries the set of instructions for cell functions. While most scientists don't believe that most cases are directly inherited, it is possible that some people are more genetically susceptible to PD. Replacing defective genetic material may relieve and/or eliminate PD symptoms.

One area of gene research involves how cells die. A process called *apoptosis* causes cells to shrink and disappear. While apoptosis may sound like a malfunction, it is a natural and necessary process for getting rid of damaged or infected cells. In PD, however, apoptosis appears to kill otherwise healthy brain cells, especially in the *substantia nigra* area of the brain. Preventing apoptosis may be an effective treatment for PD. Some scientists are investigating replacing genes in certain regions of the brain to stop the cell loss.

The advances I have seen in medical research and treatments over the past twenty years have been just incredible. Progress will continue; they'll find the answers. I think gene therapy is a promising path.
Martin, 53
Physician

Another exciting investigation is focusing on the *mitochondria,* or energy centers, of cells. Mitochondria are cigar-shaped bodies in cells responsible for "breathing in" oxygen, "breathing out" potentially damaging free radicals, and producing energy. Nerve cells get almost all their energy from mitochondria. Mitochondria have their own genes. Recently a familial form of PD has been linked to a defect in the mitochondria.

Studying the mitochondria-PD link, researchers found that a subunit of the mitochondria was defective in a number of people with PD. In these individuals the mitochondria are missing a tiny piece, which makes the cells unable to produce enough energy. Some researchers believe this defect may cause the cells to produce excess free radicals, which damage dopamine-producing neurons. Others believe the mitochondrial defect may cause excessively high levels of calcium in the cells, which may lead to cell death. It is hoped that replacing the genetic material of defective mitochondria may correct the problem and alleviate PD symptoms.

> *Some members of my support group have led productive and enjoyable lives for many years. Seeing their success has given me hope and the drive to maintain my own health.*
>
> *Julia*
> *Age 58*

Neuron Transplants of Stem Cells

Another experimental treatment for PD involves transplanting or grafting nerve cells into the brain. Animal studies have shown that implanting healthy fetal brain cells into a PD brain causes the damaged brain cells to regenerate. However, ethical issues about using fetal tissue have slowed research.

Recently discovered, genetically engineered stem cells could potentially be modified to form specific cell types such as dopaminergic neurons. These neurons could then be transplanted into a patient to replace lost neurons. Researchers predict that, if it works, they could have a completely effective treatment for PD in as little as five to twelve years, provided they get federal funds for research. Ethics may be a concern, however, since the cells are derived from human embryos. Another promising approach would be to genetically engineer one's own skin cells, grown in tissue culture, to provide the same results. Theoretically, patients could serve as their own donors. Scientists claim stem-cell research could revolutionize the practice of medicine.

Other Areas of Study

Other researchers are studying the function and anatomy of the motor system and how it regulates movement. Still others are searching for environmental factors that may cause PD.

Fighting Back

We have much to be optimistic about. The brain is a complex system, but the answers to the mysteries of PD and other neurological diseases are in there. Scientists are working hard to unlock those secrets.

Until we have a more effective treatment or even a cure for PD, we must never give up hope. We must never give up struggling to stay independent and enjoy each day.

Scientists are using my body to test new medications. Even if a cure isn't found for me, I'm glad I can help them find one for someone else. I believe a cure is just around the corner.

Lois
Age 66

Every morning when I place my feet on the floor and painfully stand up, my first thought is, "Will this be the last day I can walk?" Then I pull myself up by my mental bootstraps and tell myself, "Shape up! Get yourself together! You've got a lot of living to do today. There's no time to waste." I put aside my self-pity, the pain in my back, the shuffle in my gait. I look outside at the glories of nature, and I smile.

The joy in life comes from inside each of us. Like delicate flowers, we must nourish our joy each day. Scientists will eventually find a cure for PD. Until that time comes, we must remain upbeat and hopeful, enjoying each day to the fullest.

Glossary

A

Acetylcholine: A chemical that in the brain can act as a neurotransmitter. In Parkinson's disease an imbalance can occur between dopamine and acetylcholine, causing symptoms.

Agonist: A chemical substance or drug capable of activating a receptor site to induce a full or partial pharmacological response.

Aerobic Exercise: Sustained exercises designed to stimulate and strengthen the body and the cardiovascular system.

Amantadine (Symmetrel): An antiviral drug that can provide benefit for some symptoms of Parkinson's disease in some people.

Anticholinergics: A drug, useful mostly for tremor in PD patients, that blocks the action of acetylcholine

Antioxidants: An agent that prevents the loss of oxygen in chemical reactions.

Antiparkinson Drugs: Drugs used to treat symptoms of Parkinson's disease.

Autonomic Nervous System: The system of nerves that involuntarily controls the functions of blood vessels, heart, bowel, and glands.

Apoptosis: The death of cells by shrinking and disappearing, thought to be the way neurons are lost in the brain.

Aspiration: The act of inhaling fluid or a foreign body into the bronchial tubes and the lungs.

B

Basal Ganglia: Large clusters of nerve cells deep in the brain that coordinate motor commands.

Biofeedback: A relaxation technique in which people are taught to control some unconscious body functions such as blood pressure and heart rate.

Blood Brain Barrier: Thickly packed cells in brain blood vessels that prevent many substances getting into the brain.

Bradykinesia: A gradual loss or slowing of spontaneous movement.

Bromocriptine (Parlodel): A dopamine agonist used to treat symptoms of Parkinson's disease.

C

Carbidopa: A drug, used with levodopa, to block the breakdown of levodopa to dopamine so that sufficient amounts reach the brain.

Carbon Monoxide: A colorless, odorless, poisonous gas produced when carbon burns with insufficient air. Given as a possible contributor to PD.

Caregiver: Someone who provides care for another who is unable to care for himself.

CAT Scan: A computerized x-ray machine.

Clinical Psychologist: A specialist who deals with the diagnosis and treatment of behavioral and personality disorders.

Combined Drug Therapy: combining drugs in the course of drug therapy.

COMT: catechol-O-methyltransferase, one of the main enzymes responsible for the conversion of levodopa into dopamine.

Corpus Striatum: A mass of grey matter deep in the brain thought to help regulate motor and sensory functions.

D

Debilitate: To weaken.

Demerol (merperidine): A narcotic pain killer.

Dementia: A loss of intellectual abilities.

Deprenyl (Eldepryl, selegiline, Jumex): A monoamine-oxidase inhibitor used to treat Parkinson's disease. It blocks the enzyme monoamine oxidase B, which normally breaks down dopamine.

Depression: Feelings of helplessness, hopelessness, despair and possible thoughts of suicide.

Dietitian: An expert in nutrition and meal planning.

Disability: An impairment which affects ability to perform certain daily functions.

Dopamine: A chemical messenger in the brain that transmits impulses from one nerve cell to another, and is deficient in brains of Parkinson's patients.

Dopamine Agonists: Antiparkinson drugs that stimulate receptors in the brain and mimic the effects of dopamine.

Dopa-Decarboxylase: An enzyme that can destroy levodopa.

Dopamine Receptors: Sites on the neurons which are activated by dopamine and some of which are activated by dopamine agonist drugs.

Double Vision (diplopia): Vision in which a single object appears double.

Drug Holiday: A brief (3 to 14 day) withdrawal from a drug.

Dyskinesia: Abnormal involuntary movements in the muscles.

Dysphagia: Difficulty swallowing.

Dystonia: Slow, twisting, involuntary movement, associated with forceful muscle contractions or spasms.

E

Endogenous Depression: Depression that results from a biochemical imbalance in the brain.

Endorphins: A group of peptides in the brain that bind to opiate receptors, often reducing the sensation of pain. in response to stress or exercise that react with the brain's pain receptors to reduce the sensation of pain.

Electrothermal: The method of heat used in a pallidotomy.

Environmental Toxins: Harmful substances in the environment.

Enzyme: A substance that stimulates or speeds up a specific chemical reaction.

Enzyme Inhibitors: Drugs that block the enzymes that destroy other chemicals.

Experimental: Not yet proven or available for general use.

F

Fetal Tissue Neurons: Neurons of human fetal origin.

Fibrosis: The formation of scar-like tissue.

Free Radicals: Toxic substances produced by all cells but which can cause irreversible loss of neurons in the brain.

Freezing: A temporary, involuntary inability to move.

G

Gait: Walking or ambulation.

Gene Therapy: A method using genes (sequences of DNA) to treat disease.

Generic Drugs: Nonproprietary drugs that can be sold without a brand name.

Glaucoma: Disorder of the eye characterized by increase of pressure within the eyeball.

Globus Pallidus: A part of the brain important to motor function.

Guided Imagery: A method of stress reduction utilizing music or other relaxing instructions.

H

Half Life: The time necessary for a drug taken into the body to lose one-half of its effectiveness.

Hallucination: Perception of objects with no reality, usually arising from disorder of the nervous system.

Heroin: A morphine derivative that is a narcotic and addictive.

High Frequency Electrical Stimulation: A reversible procedure in which a particular part of the brain is temporarily stimulated by an electrical charge to reduce symptoms on the opposite side of the body.

Hydrotherapy: The use of water in the treatment of disease or injury such as soothing baths and whirlpools.

Hypokinetic dysarthria: Slow, difficult, poorly articulated speech.

I

Idiopathic: A disease of unknown origin or without apparent cause.

Impotence: Inability of a man to produce an erection.

Incontinence: Inability to control bowel or bladder function, resulting in spilling of fecal matter or urine.

K

Kegel Exercises: A method of muscle strengthening for women to help reduce urinary incontinence.

L

Laboratory Grown Cells: Cells grown in laboratory or test tube.

Levodopa (L-dopa)**:** The generic name for Sinemet and Sinemet CR, the drug of choice for the treatment of Parkinson's disease.

Livido Reticularis: A red to purplish mottling of the skin often on the lower extremities which is a rare side effect of amantadine.

Liver Failure: A condition in which the liver ceases to function.

M

Mask-like Facies: A loss of facial expression as seen in some people with PD.

Meditation: To engage in extended thought or contemplation as a method of reducing stress.

Metabolism: The assimilation and processing of substances in the body such as food into energy, or the physical and chemical processes in an organism by which its substance is produced, maintained and destroyed making energy available.

Mesentary: A membrane that enfolds the bowel and attaches it to the gut wall.

Mirapex (pramipexole): A dopamine agonist for treating symptoms of Parkinson's disease.

Mitochondria: Structures in cells that provide the energy for cellular activity.

Monoamine Oxidase Inhibitors: A general term for a group of drugs that inhibit the enzyme that oxidizes or breaks down dopamine.

Motor Fluctuations: The complications of the treatment of PD affecting the ability to move. Examples are wearing-off of dose, on-off phenomena, and dyskinesia.

Motor System Disorder: A disorder that affects muscle or body movement.

Motor Performance: The ability and capacity to move about and to maneuver the body.

MRI: Magnetic resonance imaging—technique for imaging structures inside the body.

MPTP: 1-methyl-4-phenyl-1,2,3,6-tetra-hydropyridine, a heroin derivative that may produce a Parkinson-like disease in humans and animals.

N

Neuron: A cell which is specialized to generate and/or conduct impulses and to carry information from one part of the brain to another.

Neuroimmunophilin: A substance that stimulates the growth of damaged brain cells and nerves and appears to cause growth of damaged neurons.

Neuroprotective Therapy: Drug therapy that may protect brain neurons from damage or reduce the rate of destruction.

Neurotransmitter: Any of several chemical substances that transmit nerve impulses in the brain.

O

Occupational Therapist: A specialist who provides therapy utilizing useful and creative activities to facilitate psychological or physical rehabilitation.

On-Off Attack: An episode in which a periodic loss in the efficacy of a drug occurs, sometimes producing rapid fluctuations between uncontrolled movements and normal movement.

Orthostatic Hypotension: A decrease in blood pressure that, upon standing, can result in dizziness and fainting.

Oxidation: A process in which free radicals react with nearby molecules; it is thought to cause damage to tissues, including neurons.

P

Patient Advocate: A spouse, partner, friend, or caregiver who can act on a patient's behalf in decision-making for getting the best possible care.

Pallidotomy: A surgical procedure in which a part of the brain called the globus pallidus is partly destroyed in order to diminish symptoms of tremor, rigidity, and bradykinesia.

Parkinsonism: A term referring to a group of conditions that are characterized by four typical symptoms: rigidity, tremor, postural instability, and bradykinesia.

Pergolide (Permax): A dopamine agonist for the treatment of Parkinson's disease symptoms.

Physical Therapy: Specialty designed to help regain strength, coordination, balance, walking, and endurance.

Pill Rolling: A characteristic type of tremor involving the thumb and forefinger in people with PD.

Postural Hypotension: A sudden drop in blood pressure when arising from a lying or seated position.

Postural Instability: Impaired balance and coordination, often causing patients to lean forward or backward and to fall easily.

Pramipexole (Mirapex): A dopamine agonist used in the treatment of PD symptoms.

R

Range of Motion (ROM): The extent a joint will move from full extension to full flexion.

Receptors: Sites in the brain that allow the attachment of certain drugs making them active and able to produce the desired results.

Resting Tremor: Trembling of the limbs or body while the body is at rest.

Restless Legs: Uncomfortable feelings in the legs—sensations of tingling or pulling of leg muscles.

Retroperitoneum: The deepest area in the gut containing the ureters.

Rigidity: A condition in which muscles feel stiff and display resistance to movement.

Ropinirole (Requip): A dopamine agonist used in the treatment of PD symptoms.

S

Seborrhea: A reddish, flakey skin eruption, usually of the scalp or mid-face.

Seizure: Contortion of the body and involuntary muscle contractions caused by spontaneous discharges from the brain.

Selegiline (Eldepryl, Deprenyl): An enzyme inhibitor used in treating Parkinson's disease.

Serotonin: An amine that occurs in nerve tissue and blood vessels and functions as a neurotransmitter.

Sinemet: A drug combination of carbidopa/levodopa to treat symptoms of Parkinson's disease.

Social Worker: A specialist who helps improve social conditions in the community for people in need of help and advice.

Speech Therapist: A specialist who helps restore language and helps with cognitive and swallowing problems.

Starter Therapy: Using a single drug for beginning treatment.

Stem Cells: A type of cell grown in a test tube that can generate other human cells.

Stereotactic Surgery: Surgical technique for operating deep in the brain using a stereotactic frame on the head, which along with advanced radiological procedures, allows the transfer of a probe deep into the brain through a tiny hole in the skull.

Stressor: A stimulus causing stress.

Stroke: An abnormal neurological condition in which blood flow to part of the brain is interrupted, causing nerve damage.

SSRIs: Selective serotonin re-uptake inhibitors; includes a group of antidepressant medications.

Substantia Nigra: A movement control center in the brain where loss of dopamine-producing nerve cells triggers the symptoms of Parkinson's disease. Substantia nigra means "black substance," so-called because the cells in this area of the brain are dark.

Support Groups: A group of people who meet regularly to support or sustain each other by discussing problems affecting them in common.

T

Thalamus: A part of the brain that receives information from the basal ganglia (an interconnected cluster of cells that coordinate normal movement, made up in part by the substantia nigra, corpus striatum, and the globus pallidus).

Thalamotomy: Surgical destruction of a group of cells in the thalamus to diminish tremor on the side of the body opposite the surgery.

Tranquilizers: Drugs that have a mildly sedative, calming, or muscle-relaxing effect.

Tremor: Rhythmic shaking, or trembling.

Tolcapone: (Tasmar) An enzyme inhibitors for the treatment of PD.

V

Voice Inflection: A change of pitch or tone of the voice.

Y

Yoga Exercises: A type of stretching exercise that can improve muscle flexibility and range of motion.

Young-Onset PD: The diagnosis of PD in persons under the age of 40.

Resources

Many of these organizations offer publications, including newsletters, and referrals to healthcare professionals and support groups.

The American Parkinson Disease Association, Inc.
1250 Hylan Boulevard, Suite 4B
Staten Island, NY 10305
718-981-8001
800-223-2732
Web site: http://www.apdaparkinson.com
Offers publications and referrals to healthcare professionals and support groups.

Parkinson's Disease Foundation (New York and Chicago offices)
William Black Medical Research Building
710 West 168th St.
New York, NY 10032
212-923-4700
800-457-6676
Web site: http://www.pdf.org
Affiliated with Columbia University, PDF focuses on research for treating PD.

Parkinson's Disease Foundation (formerly the United Parkinson Disease Foundation)
833 West Washington Boulevard
Chicago, IL 60607
312-733-1893

Offers a newsletter, extensive reading list, exercise program for PD patients and caregivers.

The National Parkinson Foundation, Inc.
1501 9th Avenue-Bob Hope Road
Miami, FL 33136
305-547-6666
800-327-4545
Web site: http://www.parkinson.org

Informational booklets and quarterly newsletter available. They also offer an outpatient facility in Miami, FL.

Young Parkinson's Support Network of California
APDA Young Parkinson's I&R Center
1041 Foxen Drive
Santa Maria, CA 93455
805-934-2216
800-223-9776

A statewide support network for people with young-onset PD (before age forty). Monthly meetings and statewide meetings are held several times a year.

Mainstay Well Spouse Foundation
610 Lexington Ave.
New York, NY 10022
800-383-0879
212-644-1241

A national advocacy organization formed to give emotional support spouses and children of those with chronic illnesses.

California Advocates for Nursing Home Reform
1610 Bush Street
San Francisco, CA 94109
415-474-5171
This non-profit organization is dedicated to improving conditions in nursing homes. They provide referrals to care facilities, pre-placement counseling, a consumer's guide to nursing homes, and a lawyer referral service.

On-Line Resources

You'll find a wealth of information about PD on the World Wide Web. Be sure to check the source of the information. Ask your healthcare professionals about any information you question.

The Parkinson's Web
http://pdweb.mgh.harvard.edu

Awakenings—The Internet Focus on Parkinson's Disease
http://www.parkinsonsdisease.com

Support for Parkinson's Disease
http://neurosurgery.mgh.harvard.edu/pd-suprt.htm

Parkinson's Research
http://medgen.iupui.edu/research/parkinson

Parkinson's Disease: Hope Research
(National Institute of Neurological Disorders and Stroke)
http://www.ninds.nih.gov/healinfo/disorder/parkinso/pdhtr.htm

Med Help International
http://www.medhelp.org

Healthtouch—Online for Better Health
http://www.healthtouch.com

Parkinson's Internet Mailing List

An open, international forum, providing an information exchange for individuals interested in PD. To subscribe: Send an e-mail to: LISTSERV@vm.utcc.utoronto.ca

In the body of the message type: SUBSCRIBE PARKINSN followed by your real name.

For example: SUBSCRIBE PARKINSN Jane Q. User

Special Aids for Staying Independent

American Self-Help Clearinghouse

St. Claire's Riverside Medical Center
Poncono Road
Denville, NY 07834
973-625-3037

They publish the *Self-Help Sourcebook*, a wealth of information about staying independent.

National Rehabilitation Information Center (NARIC)

8455 Colesville Road, Suite 93
Silver Spring, MD 20920
800-346-2742
301-588-9284

Information about rehabilitative, assistive, and adaptive aids.

Sammons Preston Enrichments Catalog

P.O. Box 5071
Bollingbrook, IL 60440-5071
800-323-5547

They carry an excellent selection of home health aids like special shower chairs, handgrips, grab bars, reacher sticks, sock and stocking aids, button-up and zipper pulls.

JC Penney's Easy Dressing Catalog

P.O. Box 2021
Milwaukee, WI 53201
800-222-6161

Clothing catalog for people with disabilities.

Wardrobe Wagon
555 Valley Road
West Orange, NJ 07052
800-992-2737

Moderately-priced clothing for people with disabilities.

Voice AmplifierAnchor Audio, Inc.
913 W. 22nd Street
Torrance, CA 90502
310-784-2300
Voice amplifiers for telephones.

ATT Special Needs
800-233-1222

Voice amplifiers for telephones. Some electronics stores also carry similar equipment.

Information about retrofitting your home for safety, comfort, and function.

Whirlpool Home Appliances
Tools for Independent Living
Designs for Independent Living
Appliance Information Service (AIS)
Administrative Center
Benten Harbor, MI 49022
616-923-5000

Medic-Alert Foundation International
P.O. Box 1009
Turlock, CA 95381
800-ID-ALERT

Medic-Alert bracelets for medical emergencies.

Independence Dogs, Inc

146 State Line Road
Chadds Ford, PA 19317
610-358-5314
Provides specially trained dogs for people with Parkinson's disease.

Pharmaceuticals

Discounted Prescription Medications

AARP Pharmacy

Customer Service
P.O. Box 40011
Roanoke, VA 24022
800-456-2277

Athena Rx Home Pharmacy

800 Gateway Boulevard
South San Francisco, CA 94080-7036
800-528-4362

Operated by Athena Neurosciences, a biopharmaceutical company committed to discovering new treatments for people suffering from neurological conditions. Offers full-service pharmacy by phone, free newsletter with information on new drugs and research.

Publications/Recommended Reading

Day Care, Home Care, and Beyond (free), United Parkinson Foundation, 833 West Washington Boulevard, Chicago, IL 60607. 312-733-1893

*National Well Spouse News*letter, P.O. Box 100, Little and Brown Company,205 Lexington Avenue, New York, NY.

Tax Options and Strategies: A State-by-State Guide for Persons with Disabilities, Senior Citizens, and Veterans, by B.E. Bondo, Demons Publications, 386 Park Avenue South, New York, NY 10016. An excellent source of information about taxes, including medical deductions, credit for the elderly or disabled, and earned income credit.

Parkinson's Disease Update, Medical Publishing Company, P. O. Box 450,Huntington Valley, PA 19006. A newsletter about the latest developments in the fight against Parkinson's disease.

Parkinson's Disease: Hope through Research, Office of Scientific and Health Reports, NINDS, Building 31, Room 8A16, National Institutes of Health, Bethesda, MD 20892.

The Challenge of Parkinson's Disease: Adapting to a Nursing Home, The American Parkinson Disease Association, Inc., 1250 Hylan

Boulevard, Suite 4B, Staten Island, NY 10305. 718-981-8001/800-223-2732.

Taking Charge: How to Master the Eight Most Common Fears of Long-Term Illness, I. Pollin and S.K. Golant, Random House, Inc., New York, NY 1994.

Living Well with Parkinson's, G.W. Atwood and L.G. Hunnewell, John Wiley and Sons, New York, NY 1991.

Parkinson's Disease: Questions and Answers, R. Hauser and T. Zesiewicz, Merit Publishing International, Coral Springs, FL 1997.

Parkinson's Disease: A Guide for Patient and Family, R.C. Duvosin and J. Sage, Lippincott-Raven, New York, NY 1996.

Living with Parkinson's Disease, K.E. Biziere, M.C. Kurth, Demos Vermande, New York, NY 1997.

Caring for the Parkinson Patient, J.T. Hutton and R.L. Dipple, Golden Age Books, New York, NY 1989.

Mainstay: For the Well Spouse of the Chronically Ill, M. Strong, Little,Brown, and Company, New York, NY 1989.

Bibliography

Chapter 1

Rowe, J.W. and R.L. Kahn. *Successful Aging*. New York: Random House, 1998.

Biziere, K.E. and Kurth M.C. Demos. *Patient Education and Health Promotion in Living with Parkinson's Dis*ease. New York: Vermande Press, 1997: 56-57

Chapter 2

Lang, A.E. and A.M. Lozano. "Parkinson's Disease." *The New England Journal of Medicine* 339, no. 15 (1998): 1044-53.

Rajput, A.H. and A. Rozdilsky-Rajput. "Accuracy of Clinical Diagnosis in Parkinsonism-A Prospective Study." *Canadian Journal of Science 18* (1991): 275-78.

Koller, W.C. "How Accurately Can Parkinson's Disease Be Diagnosed?" *Neurology* 42, suppl.1 (1992): 6-16.

Hauser, R.A. and T.A. Zesiewicz. *Clinical Features of Parkinson's Disease in Parkinson's Disease: Questions and Answers.* _____, Florida: Merit Publishers, 1997: 23-29

Chapter 3

Calne, S. and T. Hurwitz. *Adjustments, Adaption, and Accommodation: Psychosocial Approaches to Living with Parkinson's Disease.* _____National Parkinson Foundation, 1996.

American Parkinson Disease Association. *Being Independent: A Guide for People with Parkinson's Disease.* _____ American Parkinson Disease Association, 1997.

Stewart, R.M. *The Family Unit and Parkinson's Disease.* _____ American Parkinson Disease Association, 1996.

Chapter 4

National Parkinson Foundation. *Your Healthcare Team.* _____: National Parkinson Foundation, 1996.

Cram, D.L. *The Healing Touch: Keeping the Doctor-Patient Relationship Alive under Managed Care.* Omaha: Addicus Books, 1997.

Chapter 5

Shannon, K.M. "New Alternatives for the Management of Early Parkinson's Disease." *Movement Disorders* 11, suppl. 266 (1996): _____.

Rajput, A.H. et al. "Is Levodopa Toxic to Human Substantia Nigra?" *Movement Disorders* 12 (1991): 634-38

Olanow, C.W. "Selegiline: Current Perspectives on Issues Related to Neuroprotection and Mortality." *Neurology* 47, suppl. 3 (1994): 5210-16.

"Dopamine Agonists Explained." *Parkinson's Disease Update*, no. 91 (1998): 601-2.

Olanow, C.W. "Attempts to Obtain Neuroprotection in Parkinson's Disease." *Neurology* 49, suppl. 1 (July 1997): 26-33.

Goetz, C.G. "Influence of COMT Inhibition on Levodopa Therapy." *Movement Disorders* 11, suppl. 1 (1996): 271.

Dyvoisin, R. and J. Sage. *Surgical Treatment of Parkinsonism in Parkinson's Disease: A Guide for Patient and Family.* Philadelphia: Raven Press, 1996.

Chapter 6

"Aerobic Exercise Program Improves Symptoms of Parkinson's Disease." *Parkinson's Disease Update*, no. 31 (1993): 143-44.

Canning et al. "Parkinson's Disease: An Investigation of Exercise Capacity, Respiratory Function, and Gait." Arch Physical Medical Rehabilitation 78 (1997): 199-207.

American Parkinson Disease Association. *Be Active: A Suggested Exercise Program for People with Parkinson's Disease.* _____: American Parkinson Disease Association, _____.

Chapter 7

Imke, S., M. Seidman, and S. Loftus. "Sexuality and Gender Issues in PD." *In Young Parkinson's Handbook.* _____: American Parkinson Disease Association, 1995.

Carter, J. H. *Good Nutrition in Parkinson's Disease.* _____: American Parkinson Disease Association, 1997.

"Ginger Root Found to Reduce Nausea." *Parkinson's Disease Update*, no. 37 (1994): 189.

Leiberman, A. and F. Williams. *The Principles of Protein Redistribution in Parkinson's Disease: The Complete Guide for Patients and Caregivers.* The Parkinson's Report, The National Parkinson's Foundation Inc (summer 1998): 4-8 New York: Simon and Schuster, 1993.

"Sleep and Parkinson's Disease." *Parkinson's Disease Update*, no. 35 (1993): 170-72.

Pengilly, K. *Introduction to Speech and Swallowing Problems Associated with Parkinson's Disease.* _____: National Parkinson Foundation, 1996.

Bushmann, M., S.M. Doberman and L. Leeker. "Swallowing Abnormalities and Their Response to Treatment in Parkinson's Disease." *Neurology* 39 (1989): 1309-14.

"Diagnosing and Treating Restless Legs Syndrome." *Parkinson's Disease Update,* no. 76 (1997): 482-3.

"Orthostatic Hypotension." *Parkinson's Disease Update,* no. 64 (1996): 391.

Lieberman, A. "Impotence in Parkinson's Disease." Parkinson's Report _____ (summer 1998): 4-8.

Chapter 8

"Taking Care of a Person with Parkinson's Disease Can Be a Difficult Task." *Parkinson's Disease Update,* no. 17 (1992): 33-35.

"Nurturing Ourselves." *Mainstay,* no. 52 (Sept/Oct 1998): 11-112.

Cullen, K.A. *Helping Your Partner Know What Not to Do.* American Parkinson Disease Association, Supp. no. 9, 1997.

Evans, J. *Caring For The Caregiver: Body, Mind And Spirit.* APDA, Supp. No. 4, 1994.

"IRS Rules You Can Love." *Parkinson's Disease Update,* no. 51 (1995): 287.

Bock, G.J. *The Living Will and the Durable Power of Attorney for Health Care.* _____: American Parkinson Disease Association, 1995.

"Long-Term Care." *Mainstay,* no. 52 (Sept/Oct 1998): 19.

Tolson, K. *The Challenge of Parkinson's Disease: Adapting to a Nursing Home.* APDA Educational Supp. no. 10, 1997.

Chapter 9

Parkinson's Disease: Hope Through Research. The Institute of Neurological Disorders and Stroke. National Institutes of Hope. PO Box 5801 Bethesda, M.D. 20824 (301-496-5751) or 1-800-352-9424.

Bibliography

"Mitochondria and Parkinson's Disease." *Parkinson's Disease Update,* no. 88 (1998): 579-82.

Chase, T.N. "A Gene for Parkinson's Disease." Arch. *Neurology* 54 (1997): 1156-57.

Wood, N. "Genes and Parkinson's Disease." J. *Neurosurgery and Psychiatry* 62 (1997): 305-9.

Index

About the Author

David Cram, M.D., was diagnosed with Parkinson's Disease in 1989. Consequently, he retired early from his practice as a dermatologist. Since his retirement, he has written two books. In addition to writing *Understanding Parkinson's Disease*, Dr. Cram is author of *The Healing Touch—Keeping the Doctor-Patient Relationship Alive Under Managed Care* (Addicus Books, 1997.)

Dr. Cram received his medical degree from the University of Wisconsin Medical School, Madison, Wisconsin, and trained for his dermatology specialty at the Mayo Clinic, Rochester, Minnesota. There, he earned a Master of Science in Dermatology.

Upon completion of his medical training, he was assigned to the United States Air Force Base Hospital in Lakenheath, England, where he became Chief of the Department of Medicine. During that time, he received the Air Force Commendation Medal and rose to the rank of Lt. Colonel.

In 1971, Dr. Cram joined the staff of the University of California, San Francisco, where he became Chief of the Dermatology Clinic, and served as a teacher, lecturer, and research scientist. After fifteen years in academia, Dr. Cram began a private practice in dermatology, which he maintained until 1991, after his diagnosis of Parkinson's Disease.

Dr. Cram is the author of dozens of scientific publications. Among his numerous honors and awards, he is credited with starting the first Psoriasis Day Care Treatment Center in the nation and was appointed Clinical Professor Emeritus by the University of California in 1991.

Addicus Books Consumer Health Titles

Cancers of the Mouth and Throat — A Patient's Guide to Treatment $14.95
   William Lydiatt, MD; Perry Johnson, MD / 1-886039-44-5

Colon & Rectal Cancer—A Patient's Guide to Treatment $14.95
   Paul Ruggieri, MD / 1-886039-51-8

Coping with Psoriasis—A Patient's Guide to Treatment $14.95
   David L. Cram, MD / 1-886039-47-X

The Healing Touch—
Keeping the Doctor/Patient Relationship Alive Under Managed Care $9.95
   David Cram, MD / 1-886039-31-3

Living with P.C.O.S.—Polycystic Ovarian Syndrome $14.95
   Angela Boss; Evelina Sterling / 1-886039-49-6

Lung Cancer—A Guide to Treatment & Diagnosis $14.95
   Walter J. Scott, MD / 1-886039-43-7

The Macular Degeneration Source Book $14.95
   Bert Glaser, MD, Lester Picker / 1-886039-53-4 (Fall 2001)

Overcoming Postpartum Depression and Anxiety $12.95
   Linda Sebastian, RN / 1-886930-34-8

Prescription Drug Abuse—The Hidden Epidemic $14.95
   Rod Colvin / 1-886039-22-4

Simple Changes: The Boomer's Guide to a Healthier, Happier Life $9.95
   L. Joe Porter, MD / 1-886039-35-6

Straight Talk About Breast Cancer $12.95
   Suzanne Braddock, MD / 1-886039-21-6

The Stroke Recovery Book $14.95
   Kip Burkman, MD / 1-886039-30-5

The Surgery Handbook—A Guide to Understanding Your Operation $14.95
   Paul Ruggieri, MD / 1-886039-38-0

Understanding Parkinson's Disease—A Self-Help Guide $14.95
   David Cram, MD / 1-886039-40-2

Please send:

____ copies of _____
(Title of book)

at $ _____ each   TOTAL: _____

Nebr. residents add 5% sales tax   _____

Shipping/Handling
  $4.00 for first book.
  $1.10 for each additional book   _____

                              TOTAL ENCLOSED: _____

Name _____

Address _____

City _____State _____Zip _____

❑ **Visa** ❑ **MasterCard** ❑ **American Express**

Credit card number _____ Expiration date _____

Order by credit card, personal check or money order. Send to:

Addicus Books
Mail Order Dept.
P.O. Box 45327
Omaha, NE 68145
Or, order **TOLL FREE: 800-352-2873**
or online at
www.AddicusBooks.com